HIGH INTENSITY FITNESS REVOLUTION FOR WOMEN

HIGH INTENSITY FITNESS REVOLUTION FOR WOMEN

A Fast and Easy Workout with Amazing Results

SECOND EDITION

PETE CERQUA

with Victoria Toujilina

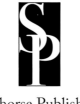

Skyhorse Publishing

Skyhorse Publishing books may be purchased in bulk at special discounts for sales promotion, corporate gifts, fund-raising, or educational purposes. Special editions can also be created to specifications. For details, contact the Special Sales Department, Skyhorse Publishing, 307 West 36th Street, 11th Floor, New York, NY 10018 or info@skyhorsepublishing.com.

Skyhorse® and Skyhorse Publishing® are registered trademarks of Skyhorse Publishing, Inc.®, a Delaware corporation.

Visit our website at www.skyhorsepublishing.com.

10 9 8 7 6 5 4 3 2 1

Library of Congress Cataloging-in-Publication Data is available on file.

Cover design by Tom Lau
Cover photo credit: iStockphoto

Print ISBN: 978-1-5107-1109-9
Ebook ISBN: 978-1-5107-1111-2

Printed in China

For my son Nicholas,
Because everything we do is for our kids

Table of Contents

Foreword to the 2016 Edition . . . . *ix*

Introduction . . . . *xv*

Chapter One: Top 10 Reasons Why Short Workouts Are Better 1

Chapter Two: Getting Started 7

Chapter Three: Get Your Baseline 11

Chapter Four: High Intensity Home Workouts. 35

Chapter Five: High Intensity Legs. 55

Chapter Six: High Intensity "Push" 83

Chapter Seven: High Intensity "Pull". 99

Chapter Eight: High Intensity Rest. 117

Chapter Nine: High Intensity Nutrition .121

Chapter Ten: High Intensity Cleansing 129

Selected Bibliography. 135

Acknowledgments 147

FOREWORD TO THE 2016 EDITION

What is High Intensity?

Take a look at the sprinter on the cover this book. Her feet have left the ground because of an all-out effort to propel her body forward. That's high intensity. Compare that effort to sitting, walking, or a light jog around the park and you'll see that the 100-yard dash is a high-level intensity compared to those mentioned previously. You can't pick up a newspaper or magazine in recent months without running across an article about the benefits of High Intensity workouts. The *New York Times* and the *Wall Street Journal* have both published multiple articles about the science and benefits of High Intensity workouts. Magazines such as *Shape*, *Time*, *Muscle & Fitness*, and *GQ*, to name a few, have also jumped on the High Intensity bandwagon in recent years, touting it as a time-efficient solution for the chronologically challenged. High Intensity exercise can be described as performing at a high level or all-out effort, as opposed to performing at a low level of intensity where one paces oneself to make it through a longer duration of exercise. Imagine going to a football field and after warming up you run as fast as you can for 100 yards, then walk back to catch your breath and recuperate from your effort. As soon as you get back to the starting end of the field again, you sprint as fast as you can back across 100 yards for the second time. Let's say that you repeated that sequence ten times. The average time is takes a non-athlete to run 100 yards is fifteen seconds and the average time it would take to walk back to the starting position is seventy-five seconds. That would make the whole workout go for only fifteen-to-twenty minutes if you were able to maintain the sprint times. Does that sound easy? Of course not! What it all comes down to is that you can work out intensely (with great effort) or you can work out for an extended period of time, but you can't do both during the same session. Applying High Intensity to strength training will involve performing fewer sets per workout with greater effort for each set. One set per exercise is typically all that's needed, and due to the higher demands on the body, workouts will have to be scheduled less frequently than a low intensity/high volume schedule.

It sounds too easy. It must be a scam.

It's not. Let me start by painting a "high intensity picture" if you will. My friend Bob plays hockey recreationally. He describes his sessions by telling me that his heart rate is in excess of 170 beats per minute when he is sprinting down the ice, and his shirt is soaked in sweat after they finish playing. Chasing a puck down the ice as fast as you can for a few seconds can be described as "high intensity skating" compared to if he were to go to the local ice rink and skate around in a circle casually for an hour. In the gym Bob will go through a series of exercises I have organized for him, starting with the largest muscles in the body and finishing with the smallest muscles. He does one set per exercise and twelve exercises on average. Each set is carried to the point where the muscles are sufficiently challenged. He moves from one exercise to the next with minimal rest. On average, his high intensity strength workouts last fifteen-to-twenty minutes. Bob usually has a few choice words for me at the end of each session, and yet credits me for the impressive condition he is in for a man of fifty-three years. His workouts with me are once a week, as he will play hockey once a week and stays active on the weekends with either yardwork or mountain biking. It is a well balanced, long term program for health and fitness. At 5'8" and 159-163 pounds, Bob has very little fat on him, his joints are his own, and he can keep up on the ice with men half his age.

I imagine you are starting to realize that short workouts are not necessarily easy workouts. Please don't dismiss High Intensity workouts as a scam or a fad. They have been around for many years, and have delivered great results. Arthur Jones has been credited as the father of High Intensity training and was developing amazing workout programs back in the 1960s. One of his most famous workouts occurred when he trained a bodybuilder named Casey Viator in 1971 for the Mr. America contest. It has been written and reported many times that Casey's workout took seventeen minutes, forty seconds and that his heart rate was in excess of 200 beats per minutes at various points during the workout. Was it a short workout? Yes. Was it an easy workout? No. It was a great example of High Intensity strength training at its best and rewarded Viator with a win at the Mr. America contest weeks later.

High Intensity or High Volume: Which is Better?

This debate has been going on between both camps for years. High Intensity proponents swear by their workouts and the High Volume people won't back down from their position. So, who is right? High Intensity is, period. How can I be so sure especially since there are many, many people who have achieved great results with High Volume training? I've been a personal trainer for over thirty years and there are a few things I can tell you with the utmost certainty. One is that a person with good genetics at a young age can benefit from ANY workout program regardless of how ridiculous it is. I've seen it thousands of times. A cute young woman goes into the gym, does a few stretches, lifts a pair of five-pound dumbbells (because she doesn't want to bulk up), and then spends forty-five minutes on the treadmill. Was it the ninety minutes she spent at the gym, or the fact that she was already in that shape before she even thought about taking up an exercise program? How about that guy with the shredded and great arms? Was his body created by his circuit of burpees, Kettlebell swings, and Kipping pull-ups? Probably not. Chances are his body is enhanced by whatever workout he does because his genetics allow him to respond to any type of training. The fact of the matter is that the rest of us are not that lucky. I wish I could spend two hours in the gym doing set after set, but I can't. My body will become over-trained and injured from a high volume and high frequency workout schedule. When I was in my twenties, I was able to do these types of workouts while eating hamburgers for lunch and pizza for dinner, and I looked great. My body was tolerating the workouts due to my youth and ability to recover. It didn't last long, and by the time I was thirty I had to be more scientific and obey the laws of recovery. The same goes for my clients. The workouts they did when they were young do not work for them anymore. Most people I meet tell me that all they had to do was skip a meal occasionally and they lost a few pounds, or they would just go out for a run and get in shape in a few weeks. What happened? Why did it stop working? Actually, it never "worked" and they simply just got away with it. And if you think that I can blame youth for great results, think again. Today's kids are heavier than ever. The overweight young adults I see today cannot get in shape by doing lots of exercise. Their bodies can't stand the abuse and will break down faster than a person who is not overweight. Have you ever heard the old saying "you can't outrun a bad diet?" It's true. Don't even try.

People are afraid of hard work. Everyone seems to be looking for the easy way or a shortcut to a leaner, healthier body. I've got good news and bad news. The bad news is that you will have to put forth great effort to make a change in your body and it won't be easy. The good news is that it won't take long. Years ago, a woman came in to talk to me about my workout program because her friend had been working with me and got great results. I told her that it's a very intense workout, but it will be over in fifteen minutes. She replied, "You can beat me with a stick for fifteen minutes if it gets me in shape!"

The pages that follow contain information that will help you reach your goal in less time than you thought was possible. It's based on science, but even better is that I have seen it in action thousands of times and it never disappoints.

Pete Cerqua
New York City
Spring 2016

INTRODUCTION: THIS BOOK IS FOR REAL WOMEN

What is a Real Woman?

A lady, a lover, a full-time mother. A woman is the boss, assists the boss, or lets you think you're the boss. She's the kind of woman who's raising children on her own (including her husband). The one who is holding down a job to make ends meet. The one who puts up with the whining, complaining, runny noses, and forgetfulness . . . and not just at work! If your biggest decision this week was which handbag goes with your red dress, then put this book back on the shelf —it's not for you. Same goes for the girls who go to the gym after getting their hair blown out at the hair salon and walk on the treadmill all while watching TV and trying to look uninterested in their surroundings.

Change Your Body in Less Time than You Ever Thought Possible

Why workout for an hour when fifteen minutes will do? It's not just about spending less time working out for the sake of saving time, it's about getting a better result because you pushed your body harder. You can work out hard or you can work out for a long time, but you can't do both.

Stop right there—I know what you're thinking: "I'll just put the time in and work out for a long time because I don't want to work out hard." Right?

Unfortunately, it doesn't really work that way.

First of all, you will initially get positive results from your long work-outs. That's because any new exercise program you put your body through will yield some type of result. But burning yourself out and regaining that lost fat is right around the corner. So don't fall prey to this common disaster we call "overtraining."

Secondly is that your body will get used to the volume of work you are doing and resist progress. When it comes to working out, that is probably the thing that I hate the most. Imagine putting in more and more time each week, month, and year and getting nowhere. It happens all the time and I'm sure that you have gone through it yourself at some point. There are two things that we should all be concerned about when it comes to our health and fitness: building or maintaining muscle and burning fat. Reshaping your body is best done with high intensity exercise and weights. Reducing body fat is best done with diet—not with hours of cardio.

Are you a skeptic? Keep this thought in mind. Imagine you were a runner for your fitness program and ran five miles a day, seven days a week. You would burn an incredible amount of calories, but provide no muscle stimulation for any other muscles than your legs. Now, add the image of eating an entire pizza for dinner each night as part of your diet. Don't you think that at the end of a month on this program, even after running a total of 150 miles, that you will get fat? Of course you will! So if you have to watch what you eat anyway, why not do the types of exercise that will stimulate your weight loss, better control your appetite, and shape your arms and glutes the way you want?

Enter High Intensity Fitness

High Intensity Fitness is about getting the best possible result for your body in the shortest amount of time. Your home workouts where you work on strength and toning will fly by and your gym workouts for putting on tons of muscle will be over before you know it! High Intensity workouts are the solution for a long term fitness plan. And when I say long term, I mean LONG TERM! My youngest client is ten-years-old and my oldest is ninety. Yes, you can build muscle and strength with this program at any age, even at ninety years old.

How Does it Work?

There are two mechanisms that are needed in any program for results: stimulation and recovery. After stimulating the body, everyone must recover so they can work out again and make progress. It's really that simple. One without the other never works and too much of either is not good.

Imagine these two situations: 1) working out for an hour a day but not very hard, and 2) working out for twenty minutes a day, but very intensely. Neither situation is good. The first type of workout is low intensity, high volume. The workouts themselves are not very stimulating to the body so your body won't change. The second workout is high intensity, but done too often so that there is not enough recovery for continued progress. The best scenario involves balancing the intensity of the workout with proper recovery time to avoid burnout and make consistent progress.

With High Intensity Fitness, we will balance the intensity of the workouts with your recovery time. Your body will never get accustomed to the workouts, and overtraining or burning yourself out is not an option.

Increasing the intensity of a workout can come in different forms. Slowing down the speed in which you lift weights will create more tension on the muscle, thereby increasing the intensity of the workout. Working a set to the point where you can't do another rep is more intense than just doing a predetermined number of reps. Running 100 yards as fast as you can is more intense than running a slow mile. In the pages ahead, I put together some High Intensity workouts that are very effective—but most importantly—they are completely doable for any woman.

From home workouts to gym workouts.

From cardio workouts to abdominal workouts. It's all here.

There will be workout techniques that you may not have heard of to increase your intensity, like holding a weight motionless (static exercise) or lowering a weight but not lifting it (negative only exercise). How to arrange these techniques within the workout, get the most from your cardio workouts, and coordinate your schedule will also be laid out for you.

CHAPTER ONE:
TOP 10 REASONS WHY SHORT WORKOUTS ARE BETTER

10. Less Time

Who has time these days? I know I don't.

Let me explain it to you the same way I explain it to my clients when they come in for a workout with me. What if I was your money manager and you gave me your life savings to invest for you? A year goes by and I give you my annual report and you have exactly the same amount of money as you did last year (minus my commission, of course). What would you do? I imagine you would fire me and throw me out of your house! This is what your "low intensity, high volume" workout is doing for you—nothing, zilch, nada. Be honest, did you lose a lot of weight in the past year with your workout program?

Any at all?

Did your strength increase?

If the answer is no, then you have to increase your intensity and be more scientific about your workouts and diet. High Intensity Fitness will yield results each week in a fraction of the time. The net result will be a better fitness portfolio in less time.

9. Actual Results

With High Intensity Fitness, you can see tangible results each week. It's very important to know that increases in strength and endurance always precede a change in the body. So you'll notice that the numbers on your workout chart will go up for a few weeks before you see a physical change in the mirror. Please be patient . . . it will happen. Research shows that an increase in strength and muscle helps the body burn more fat throughout the day at a higher success rate than hours on the treadmill, elliptical, or spin class . . . and we all want to spend less time getting what we want.

8. Very Interesting

How difficult is it to get on the treadmill or elliptical for an hour each day knowing that the only thing you get when you're finished is more laundry to do? It must be exhausting. That's why there is a new fad each year to keep you interested. How are we going to make these people come in and sweat for an hour, charge them money, and NOT improve their strength and health? This is what the big gyms are banging their heads about each year—how to suck you in. First it was step class, then it was kickboxing, then it was some sort of boot camp. My favorite is when they dig up something from 200 years ago that didn't work and try to sell it to you again (see kettlebells). Don't get me wrong—I am not against activities outside of your high intensity workouts. I tell my clients to take a yoga class or go for a walk or even try a Zumba class if you need to get out and release some tension. But don't confuse these activities with result-producing exercise. High Intensity Fitness is based on scientific principles that will stimulate your body as well as your mind.

7. Based On Science

Haven't you ever asked yourself "Why?" As in,

"Why do we need to walk on the treadmill for an hour?"

"Why not 46 minutes?"

"Why do we have to do three sets of 12–15 on everything?"

"Why not four sets or 37 reps per set?"

Well, I asked these questions years ago and wanted answers. Fortunately for me, there was someone who was blazing the High Intensity Fitness trail when I was looking for help. His name was Arthur Jones, and he is the inventor of Nautilus. Arthur was an "in your face" kind of guy that wanted answers to all the strength training and exercise questions—and got them:

You only need to do one set of an exercise if performed properly not three or five. Only the simple-minded spent hours in the gym when 20 minutes would do.

Yes, Arthur paved the way. So instead of mindlessly going to the gym and doing "whatever," we now know that results come from a carefully planned High Intensity session . . . and it didn't stop there. More articles and research are surfacing each day. A recent article from the *New York Times* informed readers about research performed at McMaster University in Hamilton, Ontario, that showed a 30 second High Intensity workout was more productive than a 30 minute moderate intensity workout! I have read many articles like this over the last few years as more and more information has come to light. Hey, there was a time when we had to rub two sticks together to make fire. Now you just "flick your Bic," and voilà!

We have come a long way in the fitness industry. The "do as much as possible in hopes that something will work" method is outdated. The more specific and scientific methods are "in." In my first book, *The 90-Second Fitness Solution*, I cited many studies to prove the effectiveness of High Intensity workouts. In this book, I promise not to bore you with too much explanation of "why it works," and instead just get you right to the workouts as quickly as possible.

6. You Won't Get Big

Women don't produce as much testosterone as men. Yes, you make as much money, endure more pain, and are definitely the more attractive of the species, but you don't produce more testosterone. Why should you care? Because it's the high levels of testosterone in your body that make for big and bulky muscles. That's why some people (both men and women) take steroids. High Intensity Fitness will make your female body smaller, tighter, and stronger.

5. With Strength Comes Tone

The stronger you get, the leaner you get. Think of your body as an engine. A weak engine will not be able to gobble up and use much gas. With a car, the excess gas just sits in the tank, but with humans, the excess gas or "calories" are stored as fat. Really ugly, never where you want it, always trying to hide it, FAT! A stronger body burns more calories than a weaker one. High Intensity workouts strengthen and tone the body where low intensity, high volume workouts do not.

4. Increased Metabolism

Check this out: muscle burns 25 percent more calories than fat. So guess which one you want more of? That means you can burn more calories than your girlfriend by lying on a beach chair while she does hours of cardio. Burning calories while doing nothing beats exercising any day of the week!

3. Stronger Bones

Research shows that strength training can increase bone density up to 13 percent in only six months. High Intensity Strength Training does an even better job. My recommendation for avoiding osteoporosis and standing up straight all your life is to hit the weights the High Intensity way.

2. Prevent Arthritis

Reducing body fat is a good short-term goal, but pain free for life is a great long-term goal. High Intensity Fitness workouts will also strengthen your connective tissues, which will in turn increase future joint stability. Having stable joints not only helps prevent injuries, but also helps those that suffer from arthritis. It's all about quality of life. With your stronger body, everyday activities become easier and make life more enjoyable.

And the number one reason that short workouts are better than long ones . . .

1. Drop Dead Legs

Look ladies . . . workout on the treadmill and elliptical all you want. Lift your baby weights and endure all the "sculpting" classes; but only my High Intensity Leg Workout will give you the shape and tone you desire. The kind of shape and tone that will make men stop breathing when you walk by. And the leg workout will take less than 10 minutes per week!

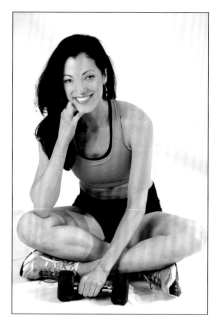

Cora Poage is a Board Certified Wellness Coach and graduate of the Institute for Integrative Nutrition.

CHAPTER TWO:
GETTING STARTED

Believe it or not, a great way to start your exercise program is with a garbage bag and your wallet. Let's face it, your old habits are not working for you (and if they were, you wouldn't be reading this book).

Time to start with a clean slate.

Clean Out Your Refrigerator

Walk into the kitchen and open up your refrigerator and cupboards. What do you see? It's all the stuff that was making you fat. It's time to get rid of it and make room for the good stuff. I know that in some cases you may think you are eating healthy, but in reality, you probably aren't.

If it's processed, made of white flour or white sugar, **toss it**.

If it has a high amount of sodium, **pitch it**.

If it has gluten or soy, give it the **boot**!

Let me guess: the only thing left is the baking soda and a few ice cubes. Time to restock.

Go Shopping for Real Food

Eating healthy and losing body fat is not about the latest fad diet or the processed and packaged garbage that's on TV. It's about real food and fueling your body.

- Fresh fruits and vegetables.
- Free range chicken and eggs that are high in omega-3 fatty acids.
- If you eat beef, get it from grass fed cows only.
- Fish? Wild Alaskan salmon is best.

Now look at your refrigerator and cupboards. We haven't counted a calorie or restricted a food group, but you can already see that this is going to work. It feels right, doesn't it? By the way, chocolate is food and beer is not. There will definitely be room in your eating plan for a slip up once in a while, but we will keep it to a minimum.

HIGH INTENSITY FITNESS TIPS

Order Your Supplements Online

No diet gives us everything we need. Maybe your joints are giving you a hard time and you need some MSM? A good protein supplement will make at least one of your meals more convenient. Most people I know need B vitamins for stress and metabolism. How about a cleanse? It's probably about time for you to clean out your system and give it the "clean slate" that you just gave your kitchen. I recently started supplementing my nutrition with high quality protein shakes, and I love the convenience and results I see. It's the one-stop-shopping that always gets my attention, but the key is to choose protein powder that comes from grass fed cows in New Zealand. Believe me, cows that enjoy clean living are better for us than when they are lined up by the thousands and fed garbage that I wouldn't give to a rat. I will point you in the right direction and get you set up with anything you need in the High Intensity Nutrition chapter.

Be Prepared to Work Outside of Your Comfort Zone

This is mental prep. You will have to work harder and smarter to abandon what I call the "low intensity attitude." What I mean here is you probably think that since you don't want to work hard, you can bypass the lack of effort with working out longer. That couldn't be further from the truth. If it worked that way, we wouldn't have an obesity epidemic in our country.

High Intensity Tip:
Listen, people slip up, it happens. The most important thing is rather than letting it be an excuse to quit eating healthy, take it in stride and continue your healthy ways. There's no reason to throw away all your hard work if you have a chocolate bar or two..

So I'm telling you right now that you will have to put some effort into these brief and infrequent workouts to get something out of them. I understand that this will most likely be a little out of your comfort zone, but that's okay. You will embrace it after a while and will not know how you endured those mindless, lengthy sessions that you tried in the past.

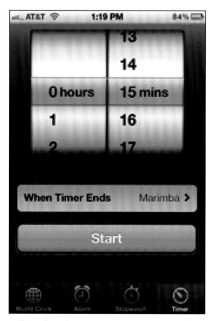

It only takes minutes to get started!

CHAPTER THREE:
GET YOUR BASELINE

So "workout wise," how do we get started? How can I possibly give you a workout routine without knowing what your current situation and strength level is?

Easy. If you just spend the first week gathering vital information about yourself, we will have the tools to make these workouts effective right from the first session. The best part is that the information gathering stage is a workout in itself, so you will get something out of it as well.

Home Workout Challenge

As you start your exercise routine, you may not be interested in venturing out to the gym just yet, so I have some home workout options for you that involve little or no equipment. But first, let's see what your strength level is.

The 90-Second Fitness Challenge

This was a featured workout in my first book, *The 90-Second Fitness Solution*, and you can also find it on my website: 90-secondfitness.com. The challenge is made up of two exercises: the wall sit and the plank. They are really easy to try, refer to the photos on the following pages to make sure you have the proper form. Your goal is to hold each position for up to 90 seconds. It sounds easy, but wait 'til you try it. Even people who are in great shape email me to say how they found it to be more challenging than they initially thought. The two exercises in the challenge utilize a static contraction protocol or "no movement." I use this technique as a great way to introduce High Intensity workouts to people who have never tried it before. In this situation, the static contraction will benefit you in two different ways. The first is concerning the wall sit. The wall sit is the static version of a squat. Try this exercise:

- Stand with your feet shoulder width apart.
- Put your arms straight out in front of you for balance and do a deep knee bend or squat.
- Go down to the 90 degree position or until your thighs are parallel to the floor.
- Do 12 reps and let's assess how you feel.

Did it get your heart rate up? Sure, a little; but the most demanding or important part of that exercise was the bottom part . . . and you didn't spend very much time there. Since it's a bodyweight

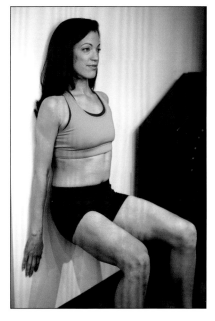

Basic Wall Sit: Try to hold this position for 90 seconds.

exercise with no additional resistance, there is very little value or benefit in strengthening and reshaping your thighs. The solution for this is to get against a wall and do a **wall sit** (pictured above).

What do you feel? Your thighs are burning, aren't they? You are getting right to the best part of the exercise and targeting your thighs with no movement. The other great thing about static exercise is apparent when we do the **plank** (pictured on the next page).

How many of you can do ten perfect (knees up) pushups or more? I know, not many. Those who are able to do a lot of pushups will benefit from the more advanced routines in the other chapters, but those of you

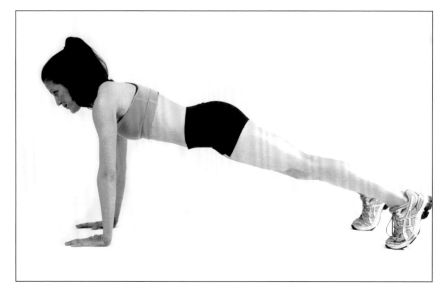

The Plank: Try for 90 seconds in this position after doing the wall sit.

that can't do many or even ONE pushup will benefit greatly from the plank in the mean time.

So, how long did you hold each exercise for?

Over the years I have found that if you can hold each exercise for

- 30 seconds or less, your strength is below average and needs work.
- 30 to 60 seconds, your strength is average but you could use more.
- 60 to 90 seconds, your strength is above average—good job!
- Just made it to 90 seconds? You are "entry level" strong.
- 90 seconds easily, you are in great shape and ready for the next level.

If your strength needs work, consider trying the home workouts until you master them. As soon as you do, get your "gym numbers" and move on to higher intensity workouts.

Get Your Gym Numbers

If you are not interested in the home workout and just can't wait to do the High Intensity gym workouts, then it's time to get your gym numbers. What are your gym numbers? Simply put, we need to know where your strength level is at on some basic exercises and apply that information to your workouts.

Our goal is to find your 12 rep max on the exercises we choose and work from there.

Write down your 12 rep max sets—make sure to keep accurate records.

12 Reps Will Get the Job Done

I have chosen the 12 rep max for a few reasons. The first is that studies show us that it is not necessarily the number of reps that stimulate the muscle, but the amount of time spent working the muscle during the set. The optimal amount of time spent on a single High Intensity set should be somewhere between 40 and 70 seconds. I have always believed that if you can spend 90 seconds on a set, then you have stimulated the muscle sufficiently and are ready for the next level. Now, at my gym in New York City, I would coach you through each set until you reached the appropriate amount of time. But seeing as I'm not there with you right now, I'll have to show you a simpler way to get this done by yourself. All you need to do is a 12 rep set that challenges you for the last few reps and your time will fall right in line with the time we need to get a response from your muscles.

Let's take a chest press machine for example. You set the machine up for your height and do a light set of 12 reps. Since the weight is light, you should be able to do 12 continuous reps in good form with no hesitation. Because the weight is light and not challenging, it will not be classified as a High Intensity set and will only take about 12–15 seconds to complete. No problem so far, right?

For the next set, you will add some weight and start again after a minute or two of rest. What we are looking for is a set that goes like this:

- You push out the first rep slowly and very controlled.
- The next four or five reps are moving smoothly and aggressively, but despite your efforts to move the weight along, it doesn't move very fast.
- When you get to around rep number eight, this is where the real work kicks in.
- You pause at the top of the rep and take a deep breath, bring the weight down, and push it up again. It will take a great effort to get it back up.
- You will need to take one or two breaths before attempting the next rep because you know it's going to be difficult, but not impossible.
- So take a few more breaths, bring the weight down, and drive up rep number 10.
- You are now wondering if you are able to get 11 and 12, but you have to attempt them because these are the reps that will give you the time

and response you are looking for. With great effort you get through reps 11 and 12.

Great job!

If you were to time this set, you would find that it took between 40 and 70 seconds or more to complete. (I have timed these sets thousands of times.) Go through the list of exercises below and find out what your "challenging" 12 rep set is on each. Start out light on each exercise and always use good form. My most important rule is to always remember to breathe. Never hold your breath, especially during those last few difficult reps, as it can raise your blood pressure and be very dangerous.

These first three workouts are to find your challenging 12 rep max weight on each exercise. It will take a little time for each session to go through all the exercises until you get to that max set we are looking for, so put aside an hour for these workouts. Once you have the information, your workouts will all be less than 15 minutes!

Exercise List:
Workout One

- Abduction Machine
- Leg Press, one leg at a time
- Smith Machine Squats
- Leg Extension
- Leg Curl
- Smith Machine Deadlift

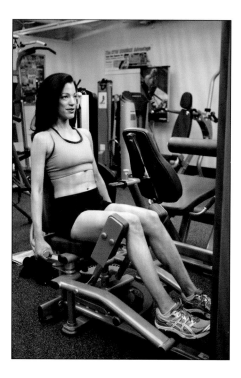

Abduction Machine

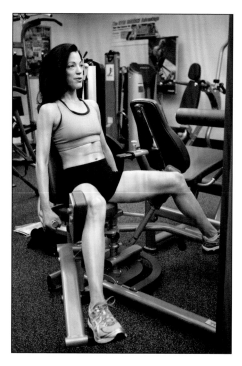

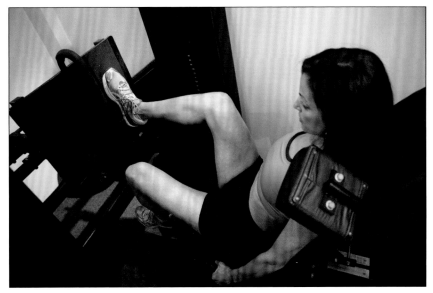

Leg Press, one leg at a time: Right leg start

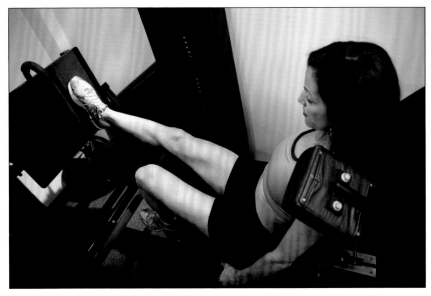

Leg Press, one leg at a time: Right leg finish

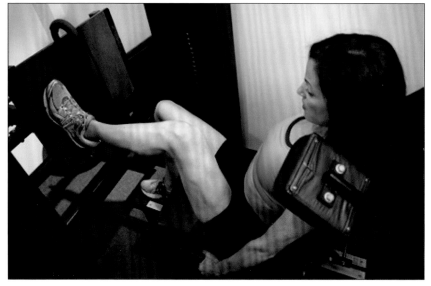

Leg Press, one leg at a time: Left leg start

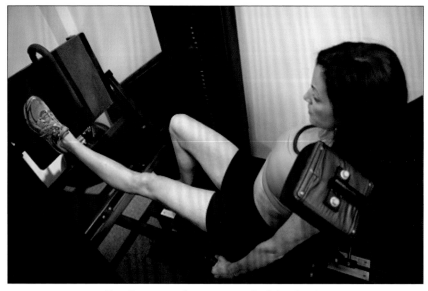

Leg Press, one leg at a time: Left leg finish

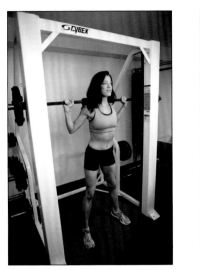 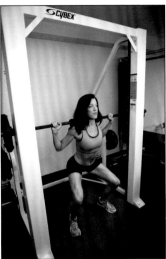

Smith Machine Squats: Start and midpoint

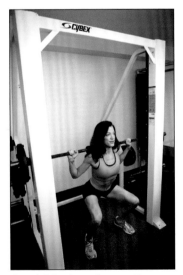 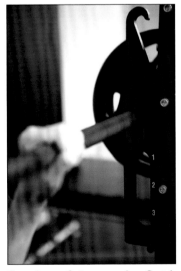

Smith Machine Squats: Bottom   Set the safeties on the Smith Machine a few inches below the 90 degree bottom position just in case you get stuck and can't get back up during the set.

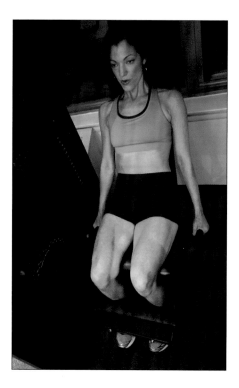

Leg Extension

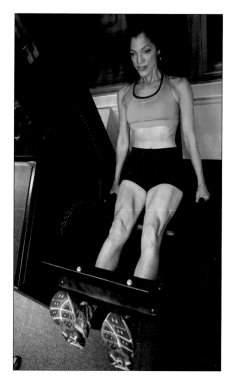

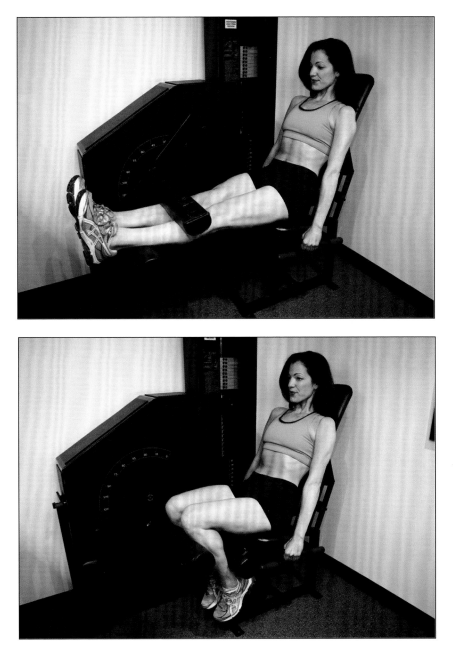

Leg Curl: This looks like a leg extension machine but it's actually the opposite. With this exercise you pull your legs back and underneath you where with the leg extension you are extending your legs out.

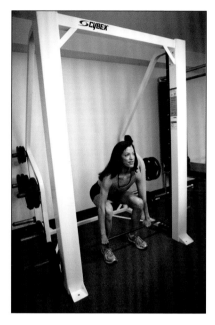

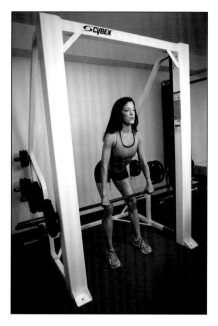

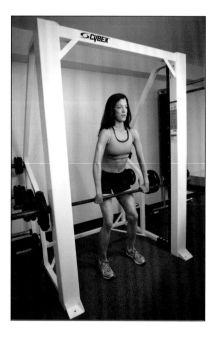

Smith Machine Dead-lift: Bottom, Midpoint, Lockout

Workout Two

- Chest Press
- One Arm Pushdowns
- Laterals
- Shoulder Press
- Close Grip Smith Machine Press
- Dip Machine

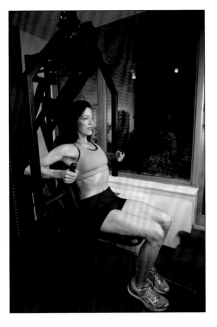

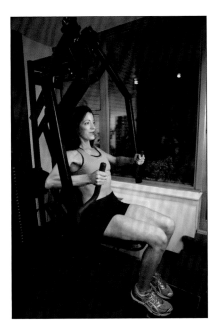

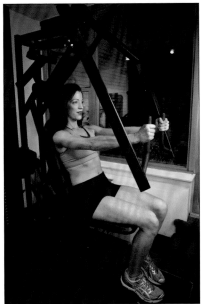

Chest Press: Start, Midpoint, and Lockout

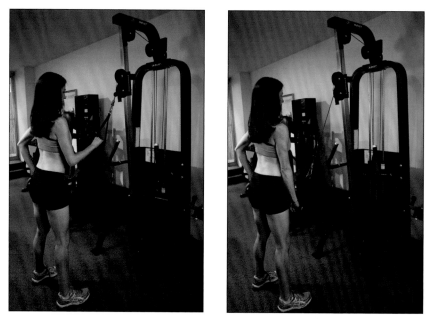

One Arm Pushdowns: Find your 12 rep max with each arm.

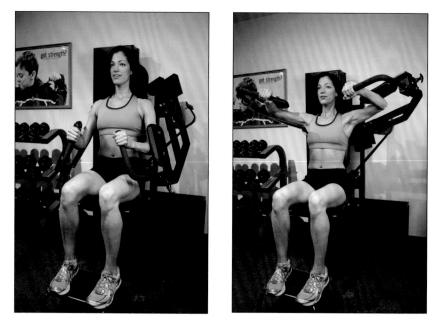

Lateral Raise Machine: Start and Finish

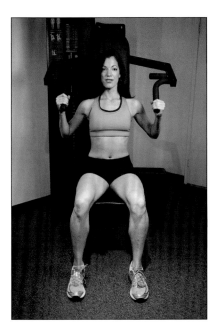 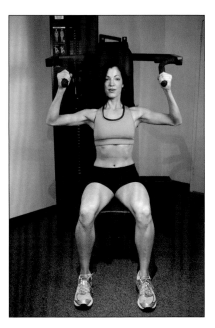

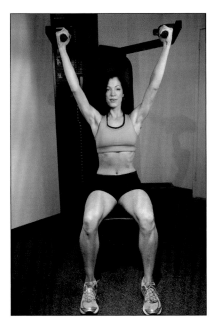

Shoulder Press: Start, Midpoint, Lockout

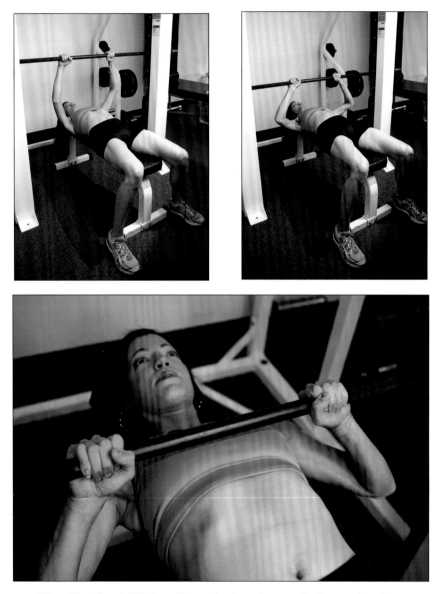

Close Grip Smith Machine Press: Set the safeties so the bar touches down 1–2" above chest level. Don't bounce off the bottom to avoid injuries.

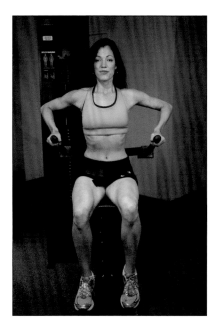

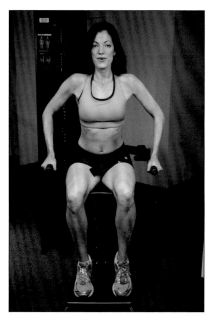

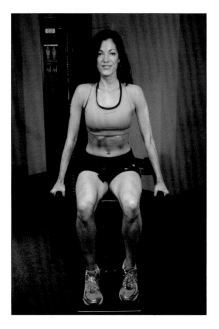

Dip Machine: Sometimes called a Tricep Press in some gyms.

Workout Three

- Straight Arm Pulldown
- Underhand Grip Pulldown
- Machine Curl
- Row Machine
- One Arm Cable Curl

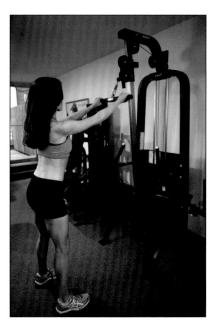

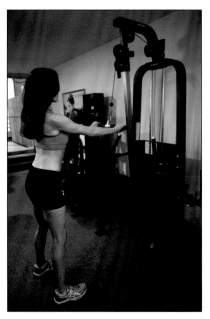

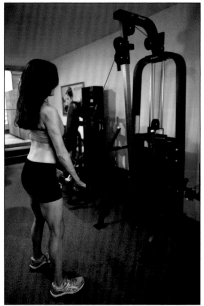

Straight Arm Pulldown: Stand in front of a cable machine with a straight bar attachment. With straight arms, pull the bar down to your thighs and return to the stretched position.

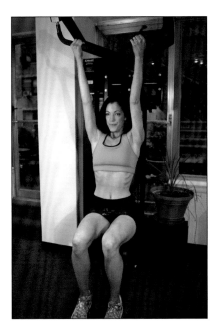

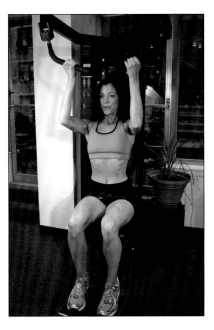

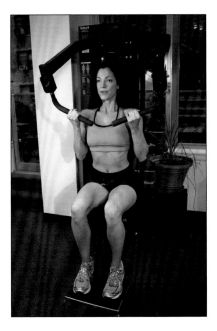

Underhand Grip Pulldown: Using the "palms up" or underhand grip, pull the bar down to chest level and return to the top.

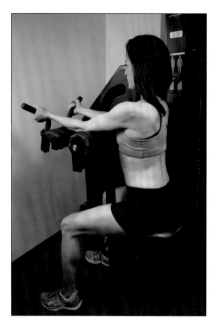 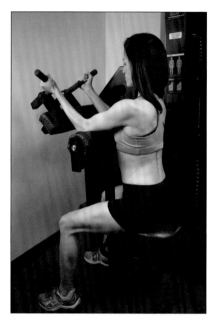

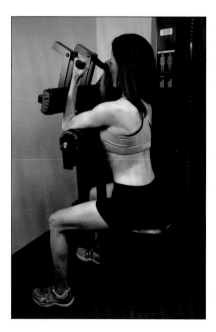

Machine Curl: Curl the handles up to the top position and return to the bottom for 12 reps. The weight should be heavy enough so that the last few reps are difficult.

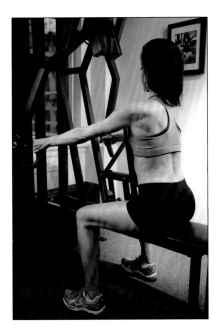
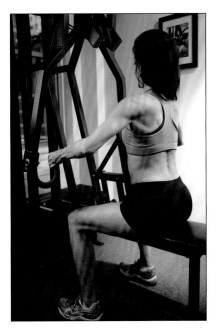

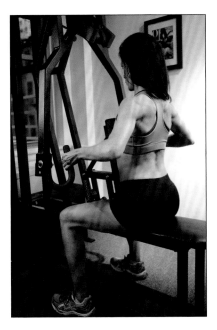

Row Machine: Pull the handles all the way back and return to the starting position for 12 reps. Keep your body upright (and don't lean back) for good form.

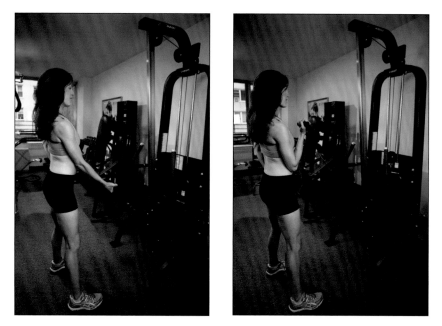

One Arm Cable Curl: Find your 12 rep max with each arm.

Do the exercises listed for each workout on non-consecutive days. Take your time and do a few warm up sets on your way up to finding your 12 rep challenge set. Make sure to record your results. You can't change your body effectively without the proper information, so write everything down. The information you gather here is very important for the workouts that come later in the book. Keep in mind that these first three workouts are basically a "fact finding mission," and will take more time to get through than our High Intensity workouts will.

CHAPTER FOUR: HIGH INTENSITY HOME WORKOUTS

The High Intensity Home workouts will serve two purposes. It will be for those with no desire to go to the gym and act as a backup workout for those who travel.

My favorite High Intensity technique for home workouts is static contractions. "Statics," as we refer to them, involve no movement. You simply get into position and hold still. I've had many people over the years comment on the effectiveness of these exercises. Research shows that both men and women can gain up to 50 percent more strength and endurance using static contractions in less than 10 weeks.

So what are you waiting for? Hurry up and "don't move!"

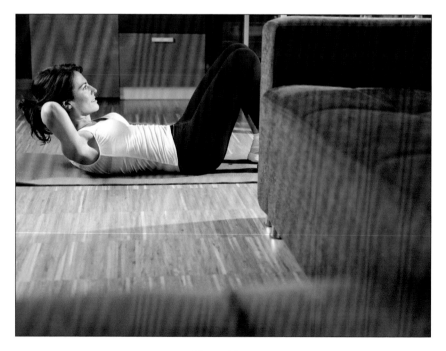

Home Gym

Home Workout Level One: Bodyweight Exercises

Equipment Needed: A wall and a floor
Number of Exercises: 3
Total Workout Time: 6 minutes
Body Parts Worked: Total body
Frequency: 3–5 times per week

1. Single Leg Wall Sit

Muscles Worked: Thighs
High Intensity Method: Static Contractions
The Set: 60 seconds for each leg for a total of 120 seconds
Description: Do the exercises in the order listed and with as little rest as possible.

Start by getting into the wall sit position, then cross one leg up over your knee and hold. Your goal is 60 seconds for each side. If you can't hold the position for 60 seconds on each side, write it down on your workout chart and try to break the record next time. If this exercise is too difficult for you then try the basic two leg wall sit. When you get to 90 seconds on the two leg wall sit, advance to the single leg version.

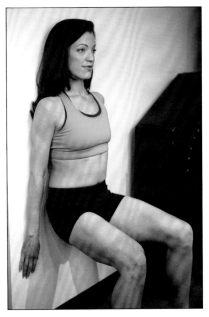

Basic Wall Sit: Get into this position before doing the single leg wall sit.

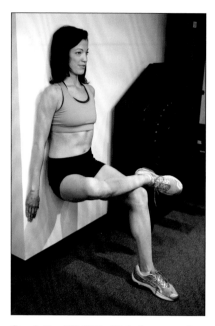
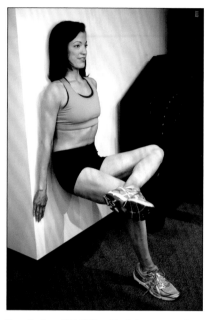

Single Leg Wall Sit: Right leg crossed up   **Single Leg Wall Sit:** Left leg crossed up

2. Alternate Leg Raise Plank

Muscles Worked: Chest, Shoulders, Triceps, Abs, Lower Back, Glutes, and Hamstrings

High Intensity Method: Static Contractions

The Set: Six 10 second static holds on each side for a total set time of 120 seconds

Description: Get into the plank position (the top part of a push up).

Raise one leg as shown and hold for 10 seconds, then switch sides to raise and hold the other leg for 10 seconds. Alternate for a total of 6 reps per side.

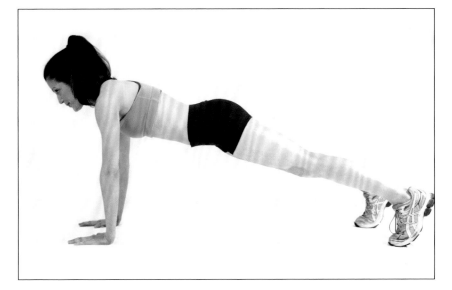

Basic Plank Position

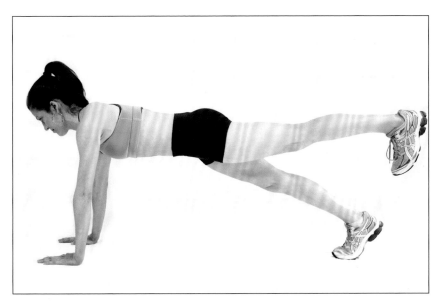

Raise your left leg and hold for 10 seconds

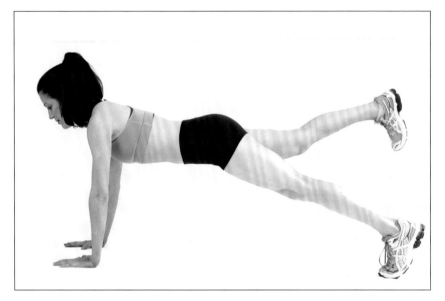

Switch and raise your right leg

3. Alternate Arm Raise X-Plank

Muscles Worked: Chest, Shoulders, Triceps, Abs, Lower Back, Glutes, and Hamstrings

High Intensity Method: Static Contractions

The Set: 6–10 second static holds on each side for a total set time of 120 seconds

Description: Get into the wide X Plank position (top part of a push up with wide leg stance).

The wide leg stance will give you the balance needed to raise one arm at a time.

Raise one arm as shown on the next page and hold for 10 seconds. Then switch sides to raise and hold the other arm as shown for 10 seconds. Alternate for a total of 6 reps per side.

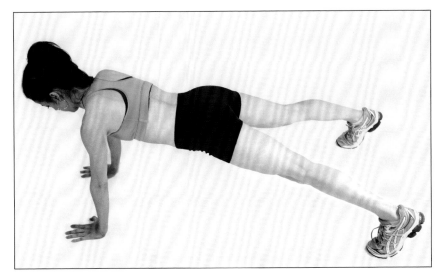

X-Plank is a regular plank with a wide stance for more balance to raise your arms.

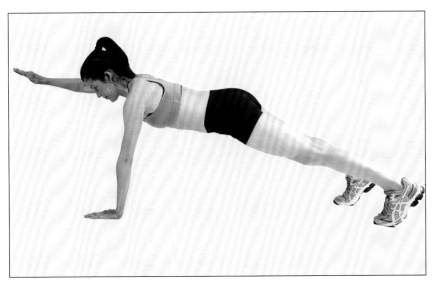

X-Plank right arm raised—hold for 10 seconds

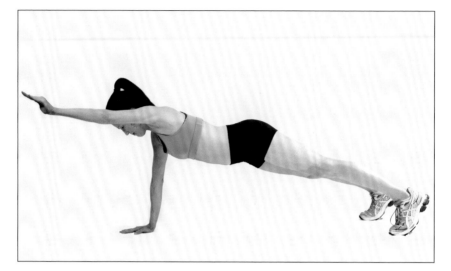

X Plank left arm raised—hold for 10 seconds

Home Workout Level Two: High Intensity Dumbbell Routine with Cardio Kicker

Equipment Needed: Dumbbells, Treadmill, or Elliptical Machine (optional)

Number of Exercises: 9

Total Workout Time: 90 seconds

Body Parts Worked: Total body

Frequency: 3 times per week

At level two, we will kick it up a notch by adding dumbbells to the routine. Remember that any time you increase the intensity of a workout, there must be a reduction in workout days to ensure adequate rest and recovery. Start with a pair of 10 or 15 lb dumbbells (and don't be afraid to trade up to the next higher pair when you master these). You will really feel the effectiveness of this workout when you get to the heavier dumbbells.

Do the exercises listed in order and with as little rest as possible.

Get into each position as shown and hold the contracted position for 10 seconds.

Start in a standing position with dumbbells at your sides:

1. Lunge left
   • Step forward with your left leg in the lunge position. Keep your back straight and hold for 10 seconds.

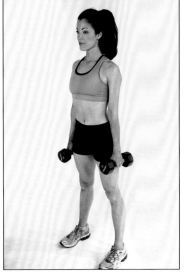

Start in a standing position with dumbbells at your sides

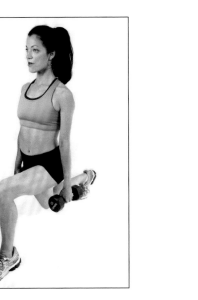

Left leg lunge. Hold the bottom position for 10 seconds. Don't let your knee touch the floor.

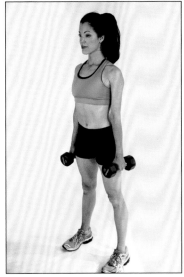

Back to the standing position

2. Lunge Right
   - After the 10 second hold is completed with the left leg, return to the standing position and then step into the right leg lunge position for another 10 second hold.

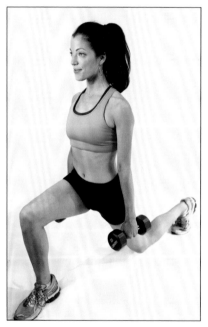

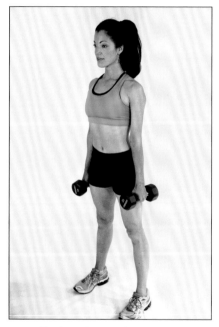

Right leg lunge. Hold the bottom position for 10 seconds. Don't let your knee touch the floor.

Back to the standing position

3. Squat
   - Return to the standing position and place feet shoulder width apart. Squat down until your thighs are parallel to the floor and hold for 10 seconds, then return to the standing position.

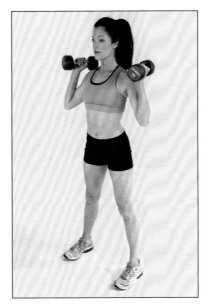

Starting position for the squat

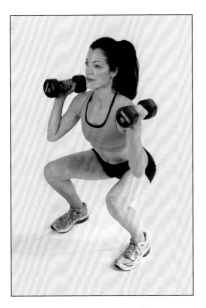

Hold the bottom position for 10 seconds then return to standing.

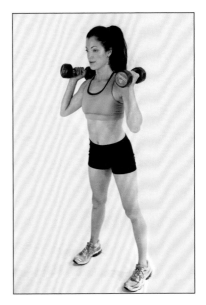

Stand back up for a moment before getting into the plank position

4. Plank
   - Get into the plank position with dumbbells still in your hands and hold for a 10 second hold.

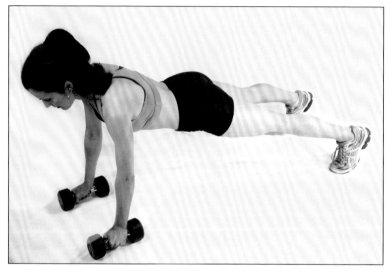

Get down into the plank position and hold for 10 seconds.

5. Plank—right leg up
   - Raise your right leg and hold for the next 10 seconds.

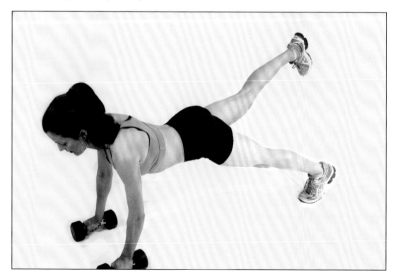

6. Plank—left leg up
  - Switch to the left leg for 10 seconds

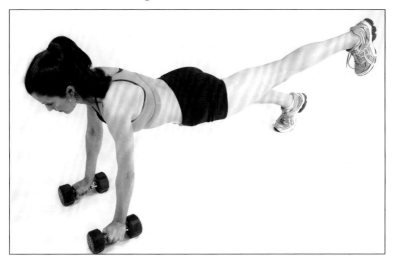

Left leg up and hold for 10 seconds

7. Plank Row—left arm up
  - Widen your leg stance for better balance and raise your left arm up as shown on the next page for 10 seconds

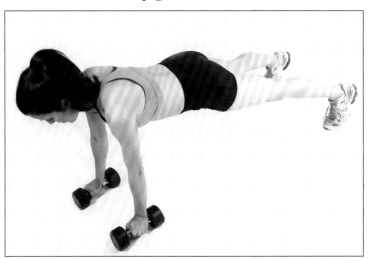

Plank Row starting position. Widen your leg stance for better balance.

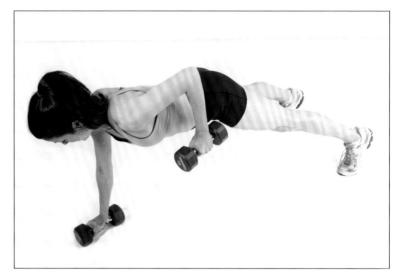

Pull your left arm up as high as you can and hold for 10 seconds.

8. Plank Row—right arm up

- Switch to the right arm for 10 seconds

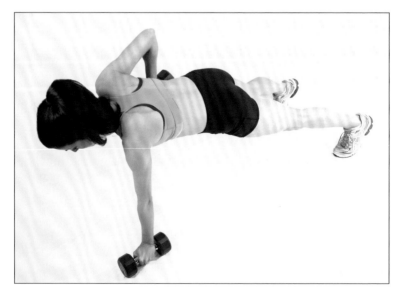

Plank Row right arm up. Again, pull up as high as you can and hold for 10 seconds.

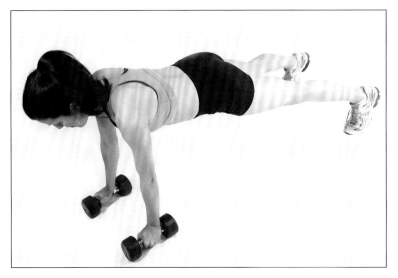

Back to the Plank Row starting position then stand up with the dumbbells.

9. Biceps—90 degrees

    • After the Plank Rows are finished, get back into the standing posi-
       tion. Curl the weights up to 90 degrees and hold for 10 seconds

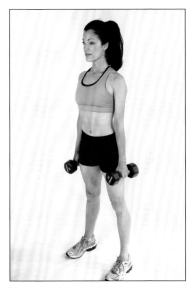

Back to the standing position and
ready to do the biceps curl.

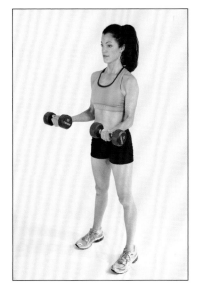

Curl the dumbbells halfway up and
hold for 10 seconds.

10. Shoulder Press bottom position—
    transition
    • After the bicep hold is com-
      plete continue to curl the
      weights up and rotate your
      hands to the neutral grip
      shoulder position as shown
      here. This is a transition to the
      Shoulder press.

11. Shoulder Press
    • Press the weights up to the
      top position of the shoulder
      press and hold for 10 seconds

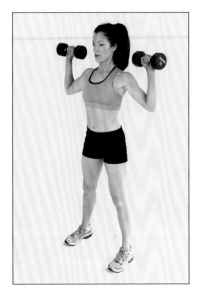

After your 10-second hold for biceps, finish curling the weight up to
your shoulders and rotate into the
bottom part of the Shoulder Press.

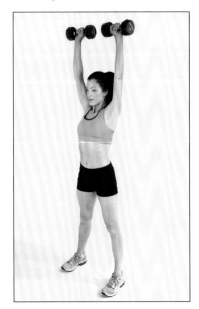

Press the dumbbells up and hold for
10 seconds

12. Shoulder Press bottom position—transition to finish
   - Return to the bottom part of the shoulder press and slowly lower the weights to the floor as you are finished with the sequence.

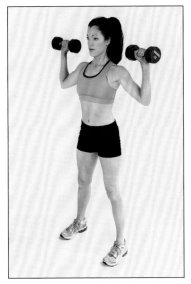

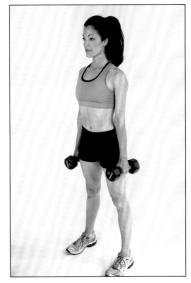

Then slowly lower the dumbbells back down to the start of the Shoulder Press.

Finished!

High Intensity Cardio Kicker

Add one of these two options to your High Intensity Dumbbell Routine for increased metabolic stimulation. Don't get this confused with the boring cardio you've been told to do for years. This is "get your heart rate up, work hard, and be done with it" cardio!

Option One: High Intensity Power Walk

I know what you're thinking, but power walking is an effective form of exercise. This is an option for those with no access to an elliptical machine. It is also the best option for those who are overweight and are just getting off the couch and into High Intensity workouts.

What I want you to do here is figure out a one-mile route. That may mean getting into your car and measuring off a mile or going to your local school track and finding out how many laps around it takes. Of course, if you live in New York City like I do, you know that 20 short blocks is the equivalent to one mile. Once you get your route laid out, get moving! The key here is to get the mile done as fast as possible. Figuring that if you walked on a treadmill at a 4 mile-per-hour pace your one mile Power Walk should take around 15 minutes or

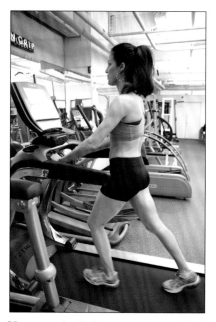

Use a treadmill for your power walk if you can't get outside.

less. Track your time and record your results. If you can beat your time by as much as a second, you are making progress. This can also be done on a treadmill by walking as fast as you can until you reach one mile.

Option Two: High Intensity Elliptical Intervals

This is one of my favorite High Intensity Cardio routines. Use the elliptical machine with the arm movement for best results. This will give you a total body workout. Start by warming up at level two for 10 minutes. This should be sufficient especially after the Dumbbell Routine. At the beginning of minute number 11, crank up the machine to the highest level. (That's level 15 on my machine but it varies from manufacturer to manufacturer.) Do the highest level for one minute and return to level two for a one minute so you can catch your breath. Repeat this for five total cycles and then do a cool down on level 2 for 5 minutes until your heart rate is below 100. Make the most out of level 15 by really pushing and pulling those handles in conjunction with driving the foot pedals with your legs.

Keep in mind that the key to High Intensity Fitness is to work outside your comfort zone and push your workouts. This will keep your muscles from getting stale and resisting progress.

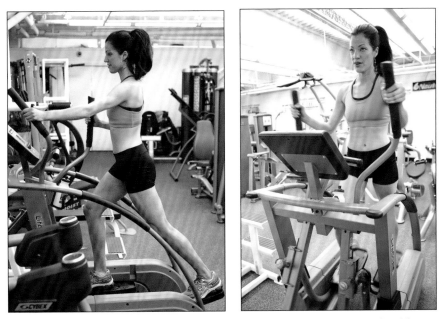

Get warmed up on the elliptical machine and then crank it up to the highest level for one minute then back down to level two for the next minute. Repeat five times so you get five High Intensity intervals for best results.

CHAPTER FIVE:
HIGH INTENSITY LEGS

In this book I have set up three High Intensity workouts for you that will reshape your body with emphasis on the areas I know you want to target—legs, abs, and back of your arms (triceps). The workouts should be performed on non-consecutive days like Monday, Wednesday, Friday or Tuesday, Thursday, Saturday. This will give more rest and recovery time for your body. Each individual workout will be done only once per week to ensure maximum recovery of the body parts worked during that session. If you get into a jam schedule-wise and need to work out two days in a row or even three days in a row, go ahead and do it. It's more important not to skip your workouts, and since you won't be repeating the same workout until next week, you are still getting the maximum recovery time. This happens to my clients from time to time, and sometimes you just have to make do.

Ok, on to the gluteus maximus and rectus femoris! (I mean, LEGS!)

After looking at the exercises below, you may think I'm short-changing you, but this is all that you will have to do. Look, I can very easily lay out an exotic workout with fifty exercises that cover every different angle and option, but the truth of the matter is that our bodies (and muscles) aren't that complicated. One "big" basic exercise is better than six or seven "small" exercises. What is a big or small exercise, you ask? A big exercise covers a large part of the body and involves many muscles. A small exercise is very specific and has little impact on stimulating your body.

Examples of big exercises are:

- Squats
- Leg press
- Chest press
- Pulldowns
- Dips and pull ups

Examples of "big" exercises are:

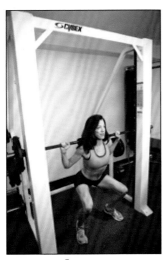

Squats

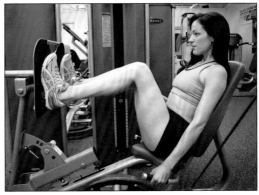

Leg Press

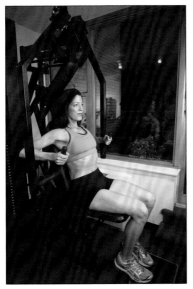

Chest Press

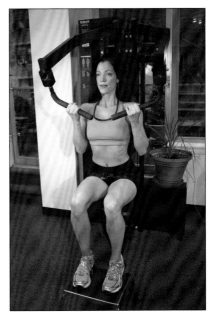

Pulldowns

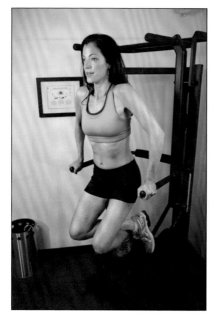

Dips

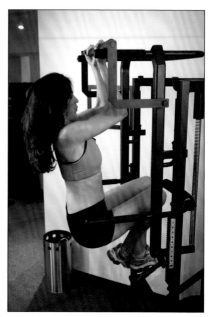

Pull ups

Small exercises include:

- Abduction
- Adduction
- Flyes
- Laterals
- Curls
- Pushdowns

Now, it's not that I don't like any of these small exercises. They have great results when used properly, but emphasis should be placed on the big exercises. Don't worry, I will still show you how to use the small exercises to your advantage.

Examples of "small" exercises are:

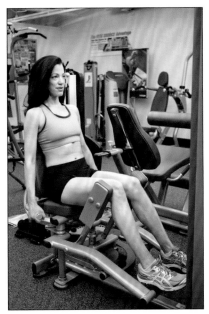

Abduction

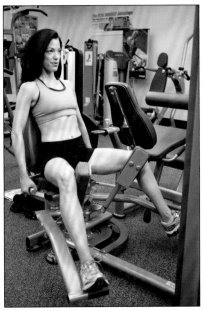

Adduction

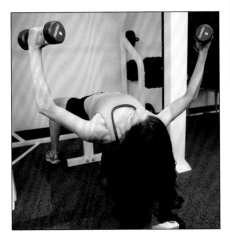

Flyes

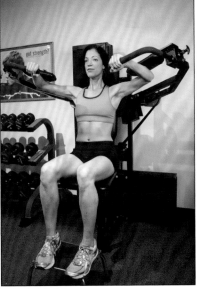

Laterals

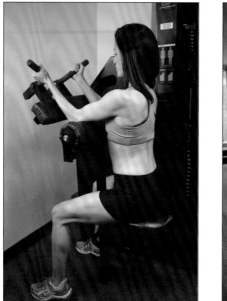

Curls

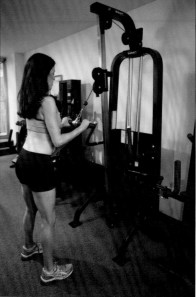

Pushdowns

You are going to work your legs once a week and there will be three different versions of the workout to rotate through. Each workout will take less than 10 minutes if performed properly.

Leg Workout One, Week One

Warm up by getting on the elliptical machine or treadmill for 12 minutes. This is not a workout but will serve as a warm-up for your legs by getting some blood flow to the area.

Move from one exercise to the other in the order prescribed with as little rest as possible between exercises. No warm-up sets are necessary during the workout, but start the first rep of each exercise slowly and controlled.

1. Abduction Machine

The first exercise is the Abduction machine. We will use a static hold technique to get the most out of this exercise. The abduction exercise targets the gluteus medius, or outer hip area.

- Get set up in the abduction machine
- Choose your 12 rep max weight
- Squeeze each rep out as far as you can and hold that outer position for 5 seconds and return for the next rep. This static hold technique will ensure that you are getting the most out of this exercise. If you make all 12 reps, your set time will be somewhere between 60–90 seconds.

Remember: All you need is one set of each exercise, so give it your all.

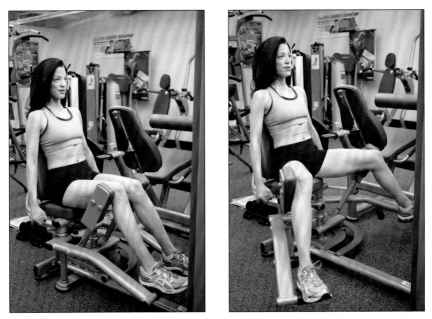

Abduction machine: This is the one where you are pushing your knees apart. Do a 5 second hold when you are as far apart as possible for maximum results.

2. Leg Press, one leg at a time

- Set up the leg press according to the settings you found while researching your 12 rep max during the "get your gym numbers" phase.
- Start with your right leg only. Make sure your left leg is safely out of the way of any moving parts while doing the set with your right leg.
- Do your 12 rep max with your right leg. If you can do more reps go for it. Always use good form and remember to breathe during the set. Never hold your breath.
- After you complete your last rep, push the weight up with two feet, remove your left foot, and lower the weight slowly with your right leg. Repeat for a total of three reps. This technique takes your muscles beyond what they can lift and emphasizes the eccentric part of the movement after your muscles are exhausted from the lifting. Doing this will stimulate your leg muscles much better than doing a bunch of smaller exercises.
- Now do the same with your left leg.

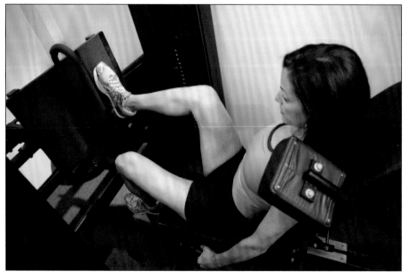

Do your 12 rep max with the right leg first.

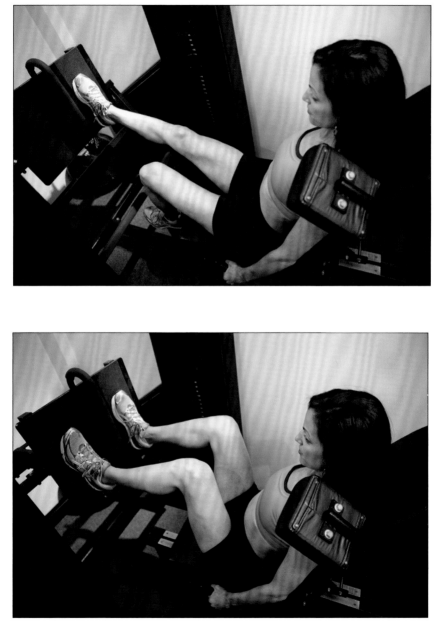

At the end of the 12 rep set, push up with two feet and then lower with your right leg slowly for 3 additional reps.

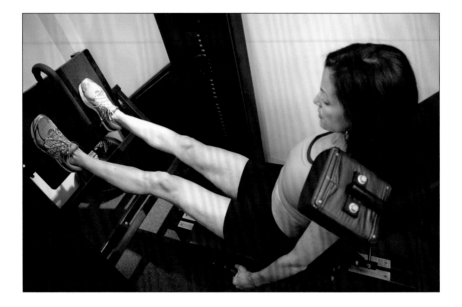

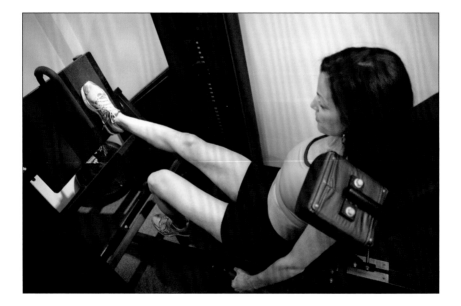

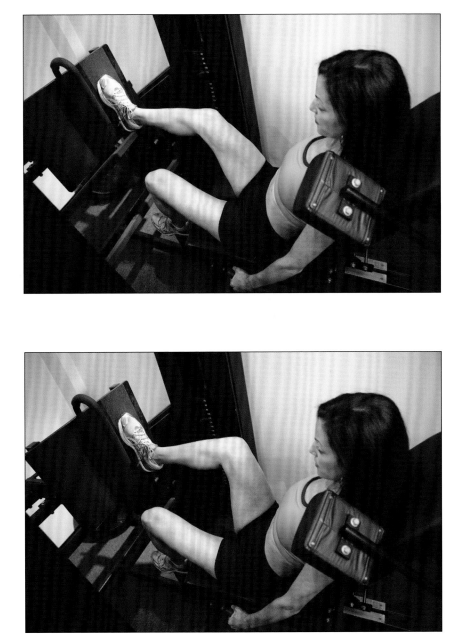

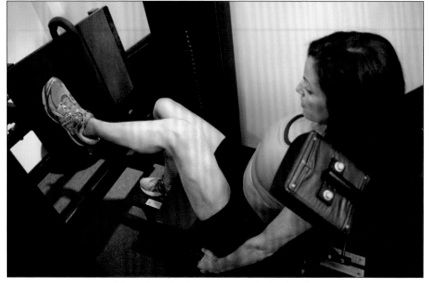

Then do your 12 rep max with the left leg

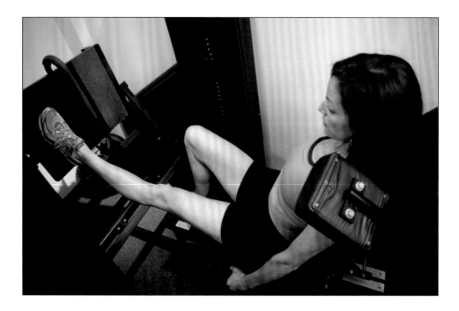

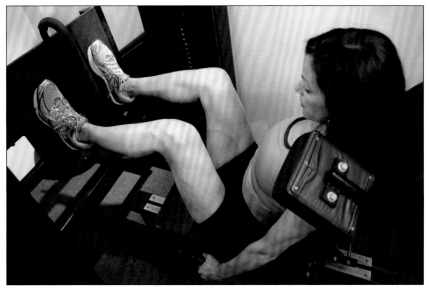

At the end of the 12 rep set, push up with two feet and then lower with your left leg slowly for 3 additional reps.

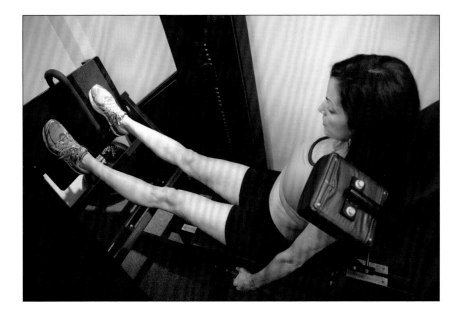

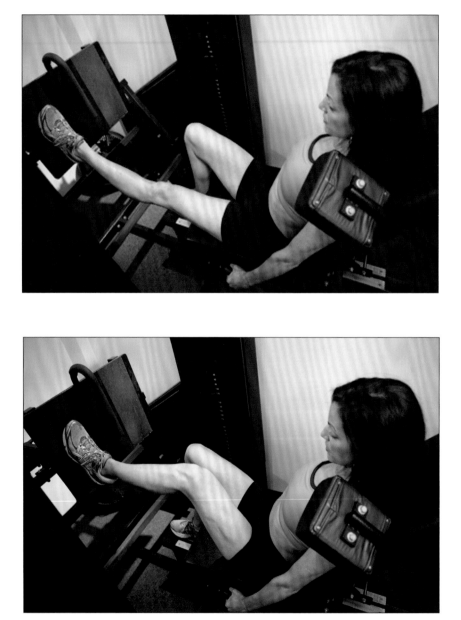

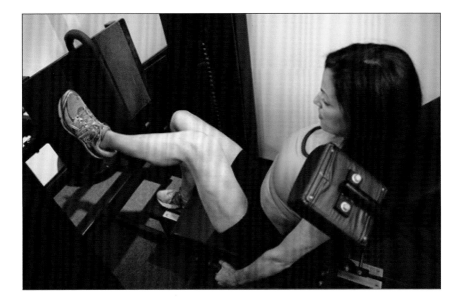

3. Single Leg Calf Raise

- Find a place to do your calf raises
- Do one leg at a time and use the 5 second static hold technique at the top of each rep, as shown on the following page.
- 12 reps with each leg and you're done! Even though you can probably do more than 12 reps in this exercise, don't do them. Instead, concentrate on squeezing the top of each rep more intensely. Knowing that there is a limit in the number of reps will motivate you to work the exercise harder.

That's it—three exercises and you are done! All three exercises should add up to a total workout time of less than 10 minutes and the best part is you don't have to do them again until next week.

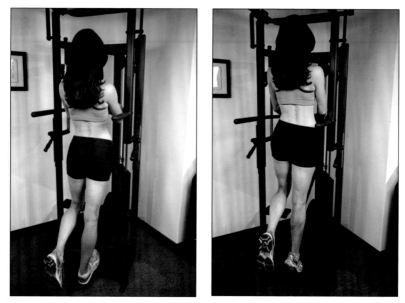

This exercise is better than most machines you could use. Do a 5 second hold and contract your muscles hard at the top of each rep. Get a great stretch at the bottom.

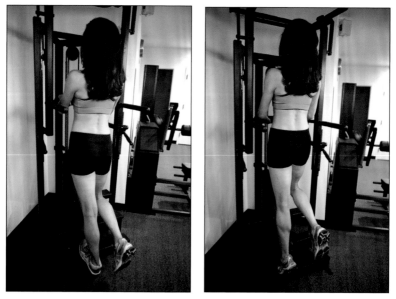

Do the same with the left leg . . . stretch and squeeze, stretch and squeeze!

Leg Workout Two, Week Two

1. Smith Machine Squats

There's no special technique here. Do a warm-up set of 12 to 15 reps with 50 percent of your 12 rep max weight. Make sure to set the safeties so the bottom of the squat is at 90 degrees. The safeties will also serve as protection in case you can't get back up from a rep.

- Do your 12 rep max set

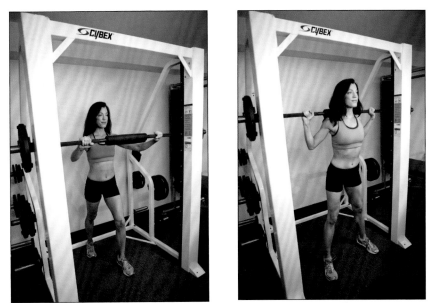

This exercise gives back as much or more as you put in it, so get ready!

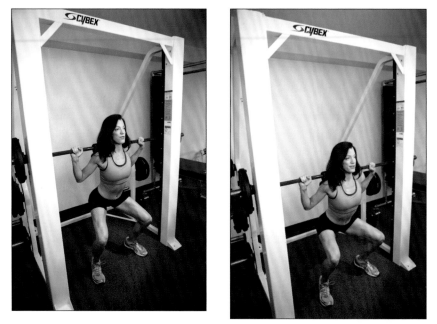

Lower yourself slowly and touch the safeties lightly (never bounce off them). The last few reps should be a struggle, but push through it.

2. Leg Extension – 2 up, 1 down

- Get into the leg extension machine according to your settings.
- Choose a weight that is 50 percent of your current 12 rep max.
- Slowly raise both legs up to full extension and hold at the top.
- Lower your left leg while the right leg holds the weight up.
- Now slowly lower your right leg (lowering your right leg counts as one rep).
- Raise both legs up again; but this time hold the weight with your left leg and drop your right leg down then slowly lower your left leg back to the starting position.

Get the idea? Keep repeating this sequence until you get 6 reps with each leg.

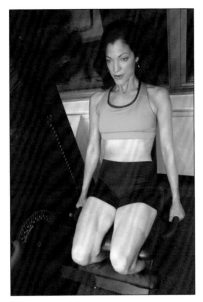

Starting position

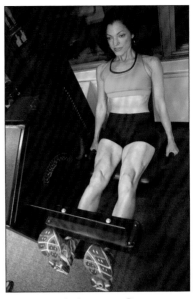

Extend both legs up. Go easy . . . remember that it's 50 percent of what you can handle.

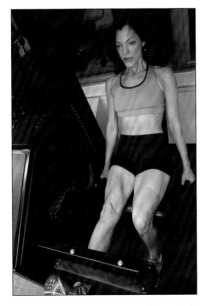

Drop your left leg down first while holding the weight with your right leg.

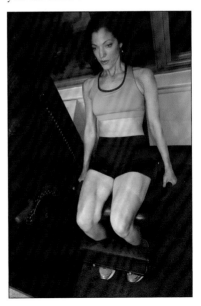

Slowly lower your right leg to the bottom

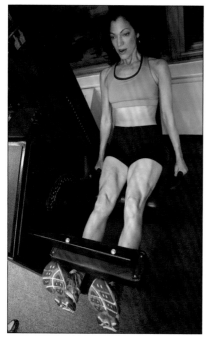

Extend both legs back up

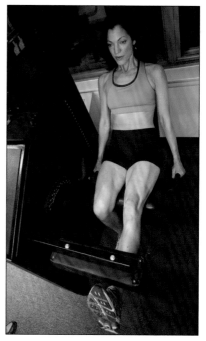

Drop the right leg down

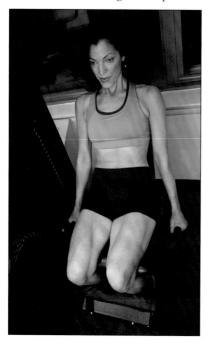

Slowly lower your left leg and repeat the whole sequence until you get 6 "lowering" reps with each leg.

3. Single Leg Calf Raise

- Find a place to do your calf raises
- Do one leg at a time and use the 5 second static hold technique at the top of each rep.
- Twelve reps with each leg and you're done!

Even though you can probably do more than 12 reps in this exercise, don't do them. Instead, concentrate on squeezing the top of each reps more intensely. Knowing that there is a limit in the number of reps will motivate you to work the exercise harder.

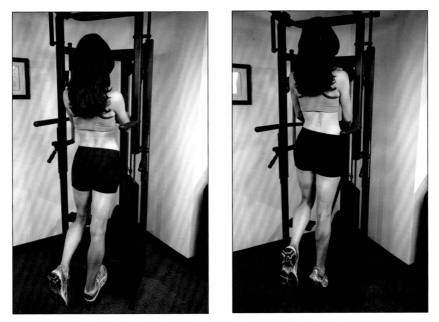

Finish off your leg workout with some calf work again.

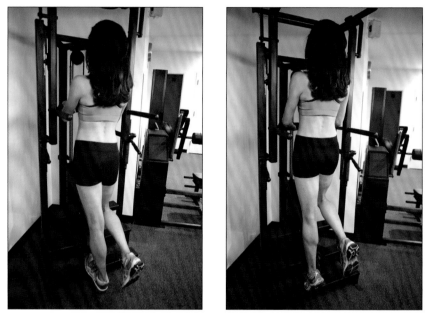

Right leg for one set and then left leg. You can do a whole bunch of sets and waste a lot of time or you can make this ONE count!

Leg Workout Three, Week Three

1. Seated Leg Curl

- Do your 12 rep max set
- Remember to start the first rep very slowly and then get more aggressive as you get into the set. Always use good form and remember to breathe throughout.

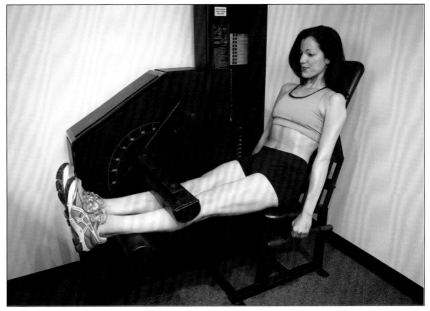

Seated Leg Curl: Just do a 12 rep max set in good form. This exercise will get the back of your legs (hamstrings) ready for the next exercise.

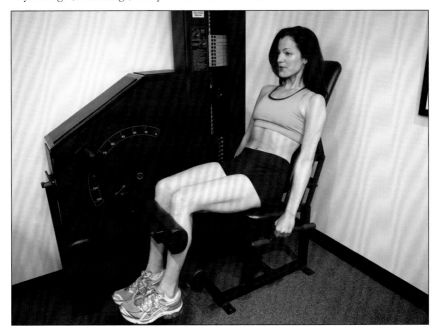

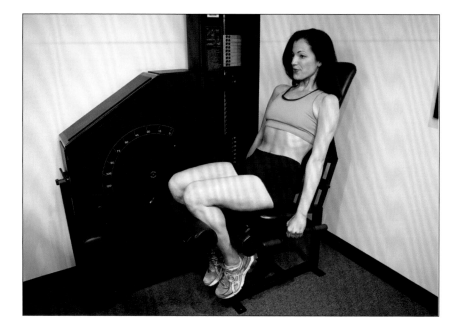

2. Smith Machine Deadlift

- Talk about a "big" exercise—this is one of the biggest. It will practically stimulate your whole body.
- We are shooting for our 12 rep max set here, nothing fancy.
- Get into the position shown and descend slowly into the first rep. This exercise is like doing a squat, but with the weight in your hands and not on your back. Keep your back flat and look straight ahead for the best form. The last few reps should be a real challenge, so give it your all!

High Intensity Tip:

Work hard on the last few reps, but don't strain and always remember to breathe—never hold your breath.

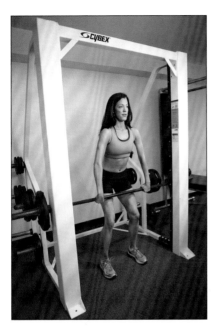

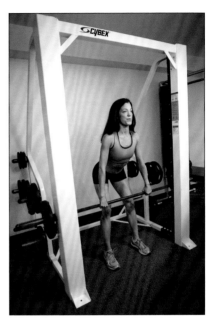

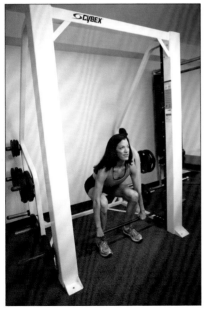

It's the combination of the leg curl with this exercise that makes this workout special. High Intensity techniques come in many variations. This one is called a superset, where we combine a "small" exercise with a "big" one to make it more intense and more effective.

3. Single Leg Calf Raise

- Find a place to do your calf raises
- Do one leg at a time and use the 5 second static hold technique at the top of each rep
- Twelve reps with each leg and you're done. Stretch and squeeze each one of those babies!

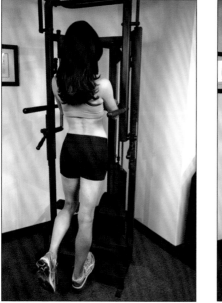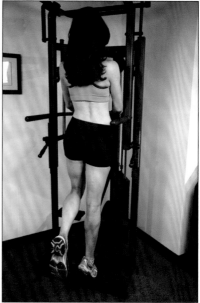

Calf work will finish off this leg workout as well.

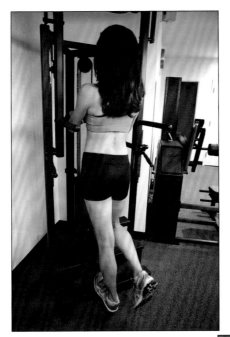

Why mess with perfection? This exercise has it all.

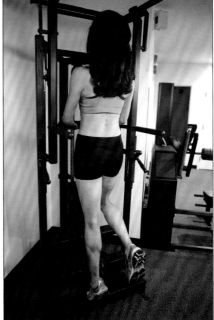

CHAPTER SIX:
HIGH INTENSITY "PUSH"

Now we are going to group all the "pushing" exercises together. I am arranging your workouts, three parts: legs, push, and pull. By separating the body into three sections, it will ensure better recovery between workouts and give you faster results. The pushing muscles are chest, shoulders, and triceps. I'm sure that most of you are interested in tightening up the back of your arms (triceps), so I will make sure there is a special high intensity technique for them.

"Push" Workout One, Week One

1. Flat Dumbbell Flyes

We are going to use a stretch and hold technique to get the most out of this exercise. Remember that there is a compromise here. You will work harder, but you only have to do one set.

- Choose a weight that will allow 12 smooth reps (not a challenging 12 rep weight)
- Get on the bench with dumbbells positioned over your chest.
- Slowly (extra slow on the first rep) stretch out into the bottom position shown. Hold it there for 5 seconds and squeeze back up to the top in a controlled manner. Performing 12 reps this way will get you 60–90 seconds of working time on these muscles and prepare you for the next exercise.
- If you feel the weight is becoming very doable, choose a heavier weight next time

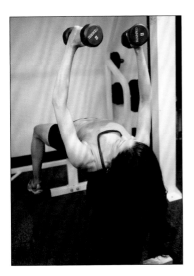
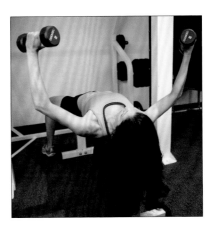

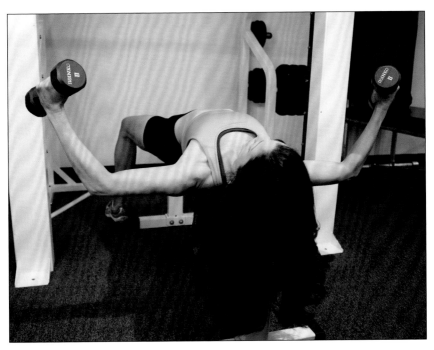

Flat Dumbbell Flyes: Slowly descend into the stretched position and hold for 5 seconds for maximum benefit.

Pec Deck—Optional

An alternative to the dumbbell flyes is the Pec Deck machine. The key to this exercise is not to let the weight touch down at the bottom of each rep.

- Get into the machine
- Bring the handles to the fully contracted position and hold for 5 seconds
- Repeat for 12 reps and add weight when the 12th rep becomes easy.

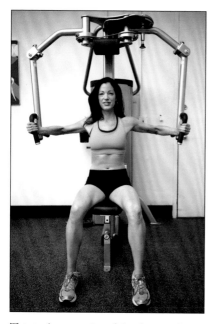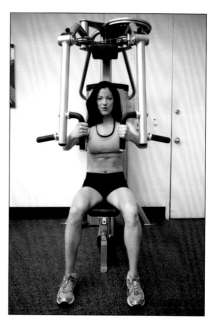

This is the opposite of the flyes in that you will hold the top or contracted position for 5 seconds. It's great to alternate between the two exercises from workout to workout.

2. Chest Press

- Get into the chest press machine and pump out your 12 rep max. You should need to take a few breaths on the last few reps at the lockout position before attempting the next rep, as the set is now becoming very challenging. If you are able to do all 12 reps smoothly and without any breaks during the set, you will need more weight next time . . . so crank it up!

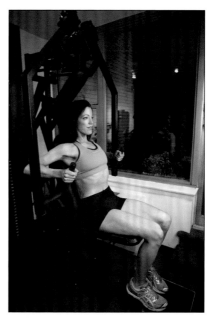

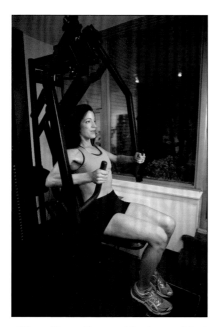

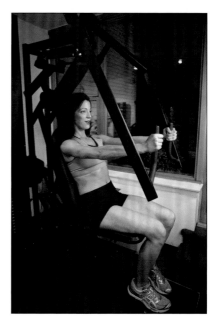

Chest Press: Start, midpoint, and lockout. Rep 12 should be a real challenge for this to be effective.

3. One Arm Pushdowns

Let's finish off our "Push" workout with some direct triceps work. On this exercise, we will emphasize the lowering (or negative) portion of each rep.

- Set up the machine with a single cable handle
- Select a weight that is 10 lbs heavier than your 12 rep max
- Start with your right hand and use your left hand to assist
- Push down with both hands, remove your left hand, and lower with your right, doing so slowly.
- When you get back to the top, have your left hand assist you back down to the lockout position.
- Do 12 reps with your right and then do 12 reps with your left, using your right hand to assist.

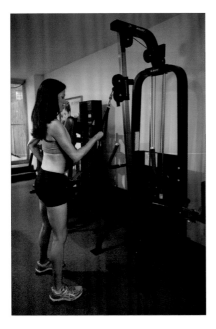 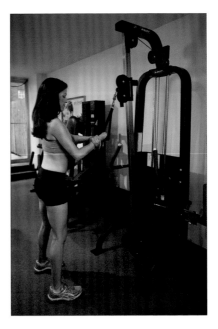

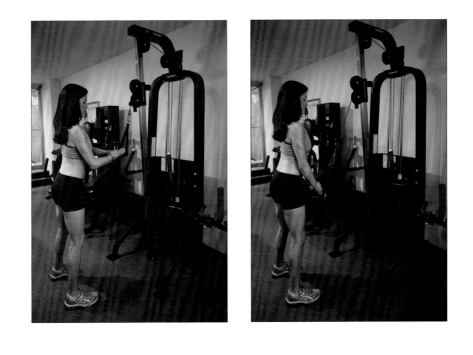

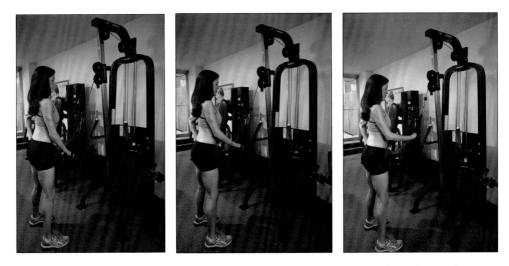

In this series of photos, Cora is using her left hand to assist in pushing the weight down into position. She will then take her left hand away and lower the weight slowly with her right. Get a good set of 12 reps in with each arm.

Three exercises, and the High Intensity "Push" Workout is finished....and just wait till you feel the back of your arms tomorrow!

"Push" Workout Two, Week Two

In week two, we will emphasize shoulders and triceps in our "Push" workout. Not only are these workouts time efficient and intense, but the exercise variations will develop a balanced look. (A.k.a. Nice curves, baby!)

1. Laterals

The lateral machine is going to isolate the side delts of your shoulders. This will pre-exhaust the muscles for the big exercise to follow (shoulder press) and make it much more effective.

- Get set up in your Lateral Raise machine
- Raise the weight to a point just above parallel to the floor
- Use the 5 second static technique at the top of each rep
- Use a weight that will challenge you for 12 reps

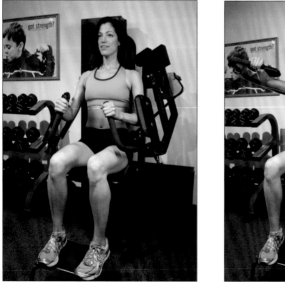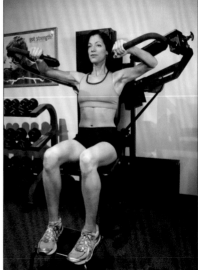

Lateral Raise Machine: Start at the top position. Hold the top position for a full 5 seconds before lowering. This would be an unreasonable request if you were doing many sets of the same exercise, so since you are only doing one, make sure to give it your all!

2. Shoulder Press

- Get to the shoulder press machine as soon as possible after doing your lat raises to get the most out of this combination.
- Use the "neutral grip" option, which is where the palms of your hands are facing each other when you grab the handles.
- Bang out 12 of these babies and make sure that reps 9, 10, 11, and 12 are a struggle.

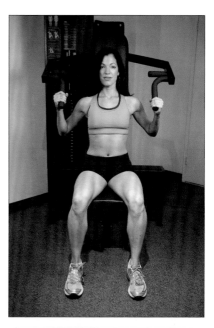

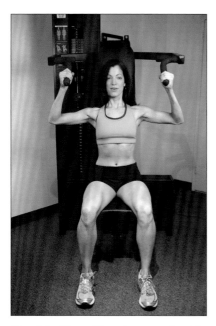

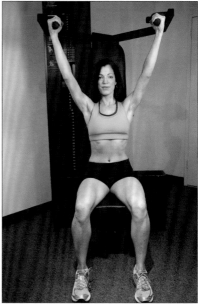

Shoulder Press: Now that your shoulders are pre-exhausted from the "small" exercise it's time to tackle the "big" one! Doing a sequence like this (laterals to shoulder press) is why you don't have to do 5 or 10 sets to improve your shoulders. You will be finished with your strength training before everyone else is warmed up for their workout!

3. Close Grip Smith Machine Press

This exercise will tie the whole workout together. It's a great movement for all the pushing muscles (chest, shoulders, and triceps).

- Set up the Smith Machine with a flat bench.
- Set the safeties so that the bar will not touch your chest and instead stop about 1–2" above. Since there is more muscle activation at the bottom of this movement than in the lockout position, we will use the 3 short, 1 long method to emphasize the lower, more intense portion of the exercise.
- Lower the first rep very slowly.
- Barely touch the safeties. Never bounce or bang into them.
- Push halfway up for 3 short reps and then lock out the fourth.
- That whole sequence counts as *one* rep: 3 short and 1 long = one.
- Do a 12 rep max set.

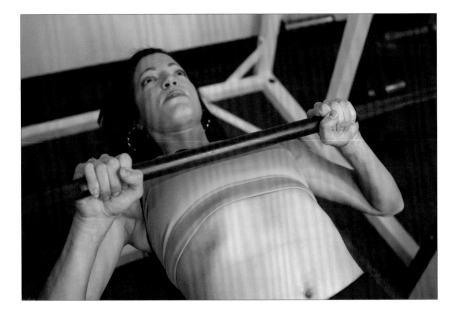

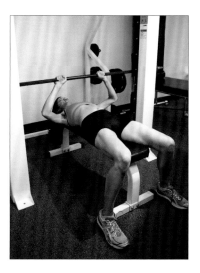

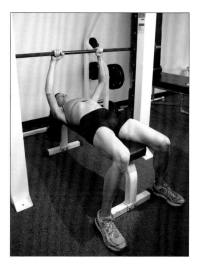

Do three short reps before locking out your arms.

Lockout the 4th push and count the whole sequence as ONE rep.
3 short and 1 lockout = one rep.

"Push" Workout Three, Week Three

Okay, let's stop playing around and get to some serious work! The last two push workouts are very tough and effective, but I have saved the most intense for last. This workout consists of just *one* exercise that will exploit all of the different ways to get deep into the muscle fibers. Positive, Static, and Negative strength.

1. Dips or Dip Machine

If you are strong enough to do a set of dips, then just jump up there and go right ahead. Your goal is 12 reps while lowering yourself to the 90 degree arm position. If you are able to get to 12 reps easily, your next step is to lower yourself slowly over 4 seconds and push up more aggressively.

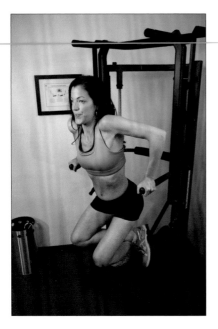

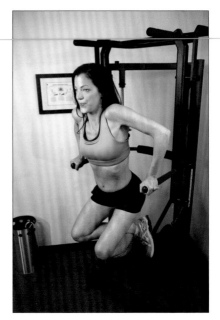

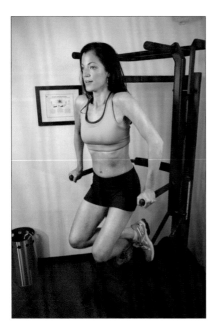

Dips: If you can do a set of Dips, then you are amazing! If you can't, keep increasing your strength on the other versions of the dip until you can get back here and crank out some reps.

If you are unable to do Dips with your bodyweight, then find its equivalent in the gym. Every gym these days has either a machine that will assist you with chin ups and dips or an individual dip machine. Whichever you choose, do a 12 rep max set then go immediately to a set of dip bars so you can do the next version of our High Intensity exercise.

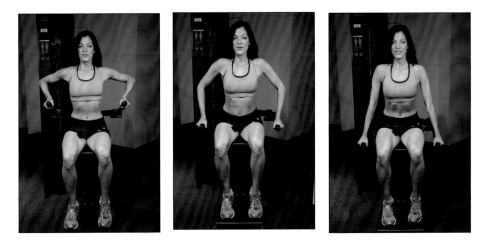

Dip Machine: Increase your strength with this exercise until you are strong enough to do a set of bodyweight dips.

2. Static Dips

- Get into the top part of this exercise.
- Bend your elbows slightly and hold that position for up to 30 seconds. You can time yourself with a watch, stopwatch, or cell phone. After you complete the 30 second hold, step down and take a short break before doing the last version of this exercise.

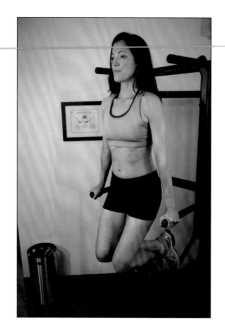

Static Dips: Jump up into position and don't move! Your goal is to hold for 30 seconds and then lower slowly. Rest only a minute before the next High Intensity version of this exercise.

3. Negative Only Dips

- Getting back up on the same dip bar into the top position, you will lower yourself as slowly as possible for three reps total with your goal being a minimum of 40 seconds and a maximum of 60 seconds in three reps.
- After you lower yourself for the first rep, put your feet on the floor, take a deep breath, and climb back up into the top position. Again lower yourself as slowly as possible and try to accumulate as many seconds as you can.
- Do the third rep the same way. You will most likely notice that you achieved the most time on the first rep, a little less on the second, and much less on the third. That's a good thing! It means that you were stimulating the muscles effectively.
- Record your progress and start the push cycle over again next week.

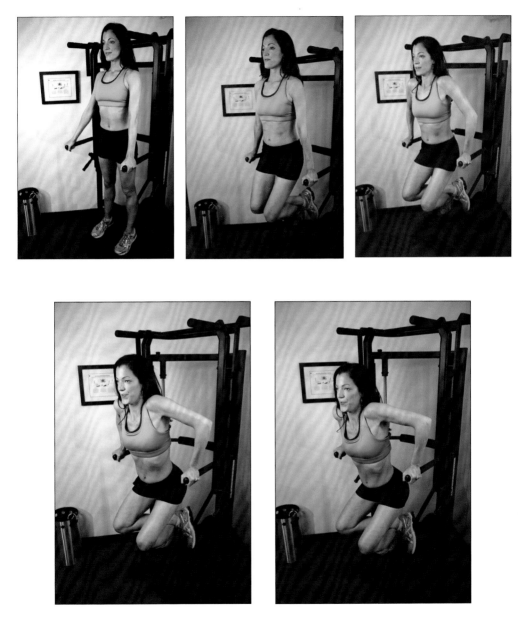

This time you will emphasize the lowering part of the exercise. Climb up into position and lower yourself as slowly as possible. Your goal is to lower yourself in 20 seconds for each of the three reps.

CHAPTER SEVEN: HIGH INTENSITY "PULL"

The "pulling" muscles are basically the muscles of the back and biceps, but with my High Intensity workouts, many more muscles usually get involved. When I give these workouts to my clients, the ladies comment on how good their abs feel the next day in addition to the immediate effect the workout has on their arms. Remember the standard set by Linda Hamilton in the *Terminator* movie? "Linda Hamilton arms" has been my biggest request for years, and now I'm going to show you how to get them!

"Pull" Workout One, Week One

This first workout will emphasize the muscles of the upper back. We will pre-exhaust the back muscles with two exercises and then finish off the biceps, which will already be fatigued from the pulldown exercise.

1. Straight Arm Pulldown

This exercise is much better than doing pullovers with a dumbbell because there is tension on the muscles at the bottom of the exercise where with the dumbbell pullover there is none.

- Stand in front of a cable machine that has a short straight bar attached.
- Grip the handles and take two steps back.
- From a fully stretched position and arms only slightly bent, bring your hands down to your thighs.
- Use the 5 second hold technique to increase the effectiveness of the movement.
- Do a 12 rep max on this set and get over to the pulldown machine ASAP.

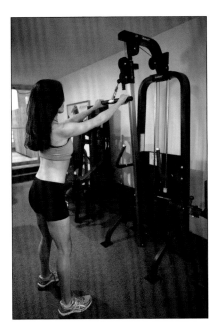 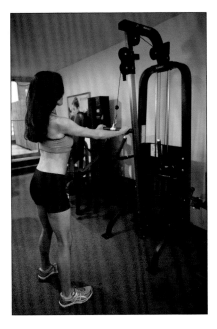

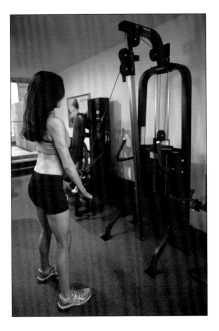

This is a great exercise that will work your back, triceps, and ab muscles. It will also set you up for the "big" exercise up next.

2. Underhand Grip Pulldown

- Select the weight that will challenge you for 12 reps.
- Use a shoulder width underhand grip.
- Get into position with arms stretched.
- Pull down slowly on the first rep, holding at the bottom for a count of 5 and then back up. Get more aggressive with each rep but make sure you hold for a count of 5 at the bottom.
- Keep your back flat by sitting up straight throughout the set and remember to breathe even when the reps get tough.

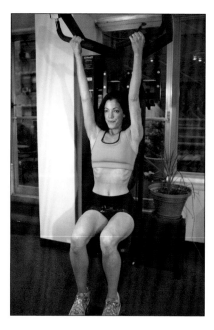
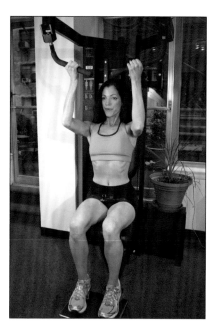

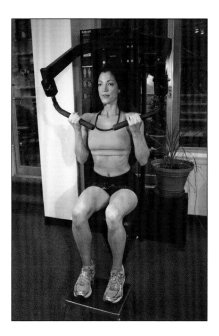

Do a challenging 12 rep set after the Straight Arm Pulldowns.

3. Machine Curl

- The machine curl will isolate the biceps better than a dumbbell or barbell. It will also encourage better form when the set gets difficult.
- Do a 12 rep max set here and use the 5 second hold technique in the contracted position.
- One set of three different exercises, and you are finished.

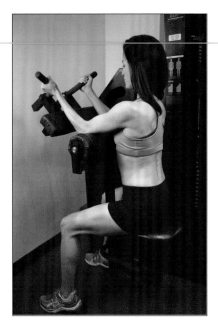 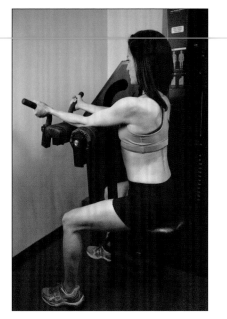

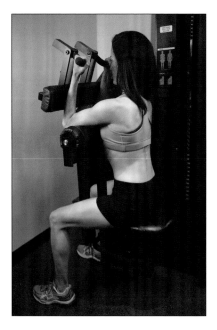

Finish off your "Pull" workout with some direct bicep work. Because your biceps are fatigued from the previous exercise, you will only need ONE good set to put on the finishing touches.

"Pull" Workout Two, Week Two

I'm giving you the most intense workout of the "Pull" cycle in week two. Why? Better to get this over with sooner rather than later. This is going to be like the exercise that was in the "Push" workout, so you will recognize the workout right away.

1. Underhand Grip Chins or Pulldowns

The day that you can do an underhand chin up on your own will be the single most rewarding accomplishment in your workouts. I get the most satisfaction when a woman tells me that she thought she would never be able to do one of these AFTER she does one.

- Option One: Hang from a chin up bar with an underhand grip and pull yourself up until your chin gets over the bar for as many reps as you can. If you can do one rep this time, then your goal will be two reps next time. If you can't do any chin ups, go straight to option two.
- Option Two: Do a 12 rep max set on the underhand grip pulldown bar, but try to increase the weight as often as possible to get strong enough for Option One!

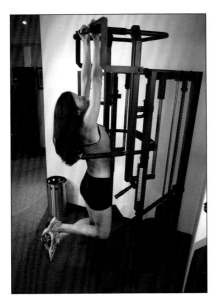 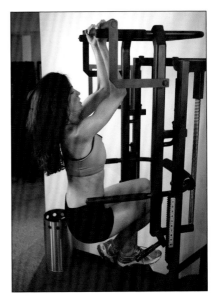

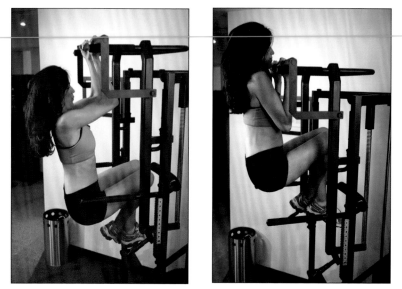

You know you are strong and in good shape if you can do a chin up! The underhand grip is the stronger option and will get you there faster.

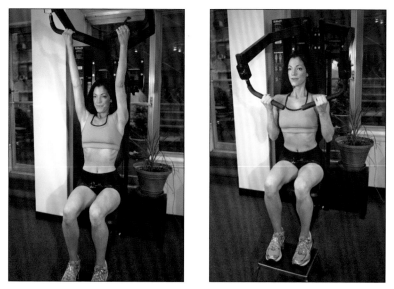

Use the Pulldown exercise if you can't do chin ups yet. Keep getting stronger at the Pulldowns until you can do the chins. Your first chin up is very empowering!

2. Static Hold Chins

Even if you can't do a single chin up, you will be able to hold the top position for some time.

- Climb up into the top position of the chin up and attempt to hold for 30 seconds.
- Keep your knees up at a 90 degree position so you can work your abs as well.
- Lower yourself carefully after you reach 30 seconds or can't hold anymore.

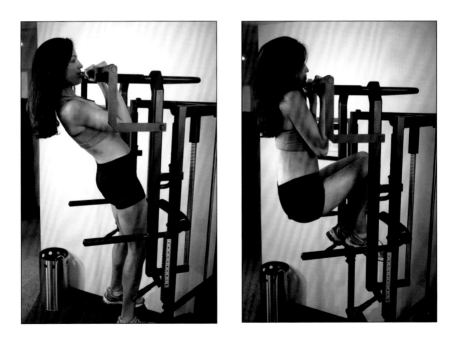

Jump up and hold! Your goal is to do so for 30 seconds.

3. Negative Only Chins

Now that you have weakened your muscles positively (the lifting phase) and statically (the holding phase), we are going to finish them off with a negative only strength exercise, which means that all you have to do is lower the weight (or yourself). No lifting.

- For this set of underhand grip chins only 3 reps are required.
- Climb up to the top position and hold yourself statically just like in the last set. This time, only hold for 5 seconds and then start to lower yourself, keeping your knees up to work your abs.
- Go as slow as possible . . . and I mean really fight it all the way down. When you reach the fully stretched position at the bottom, hang there for a few seconds and then put your feet down. Rest for a minute and check your time.

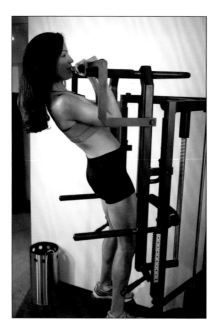 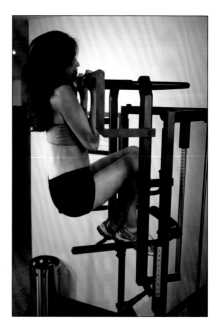

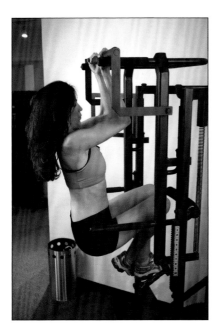

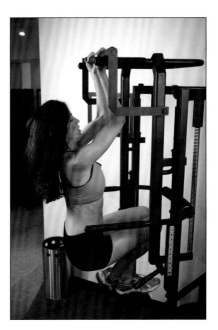

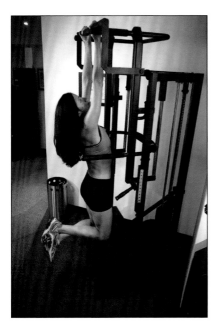

Just do the "lowering" part this time. Jump up and lower yourself as slowly as you can. Your goal is 30 seconds each rep for three "lowering only" reps.

How many seconds did it take you to hold and lower? Make a quick note of it and then climb back up and do it again.

Your goal is to be able to do three negative only reps for 30 seconds each. No matter how strong you get, this workout will always be a challenge and deliver results.

"Pull" Workout Three, Week Three

Workout Three of this cycle is a little less intense than last week's workout but no less effective. We will be targeting the mid back, rear delts (back of the shoulders) and biceps in a different way. The great thing about all of these High Intensity workouts is that your body will never get accustomed to any one workout and the variety will keep you mentally motivated.

1. Underhand Grip Bodyweight Row

- Use the Smith Machine for this exercise. Get into the position shown on the next page where you are hanging by your arms with an underhand grip. We are using the underhand grip for all these pulling exercises because it is the strongest grip out of all the options and will give you the greatest and fastest results. Make sure your hips are up and your legs are at a 90 degree position to start.
- Pull yourself up to the bar or as high as you can go. Try to arch your back a little as you go up. This will increase the contraction of the mid-back muscles.
- Aim for 12 reps. If you are able to get 12 reps with no problem, feel free to torture yourself more by holding the top position for 5 seconds; this will ensure that you get the appropriate amount of time on the exercise. Remember that if you were working with me at my gym, I would probably make you hold it a little longer.

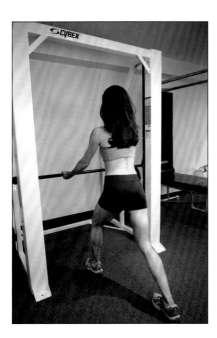

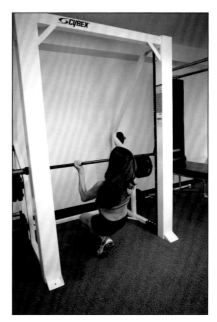

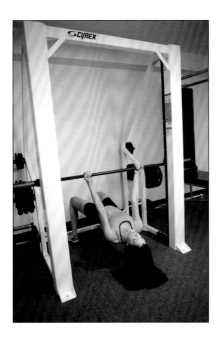

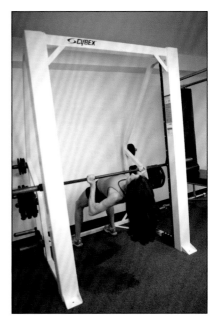

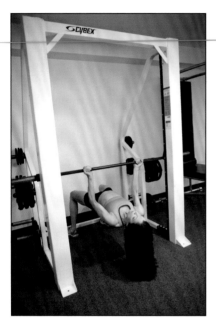

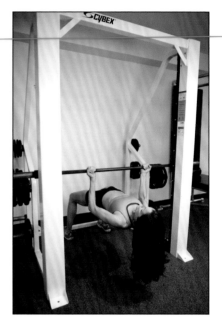

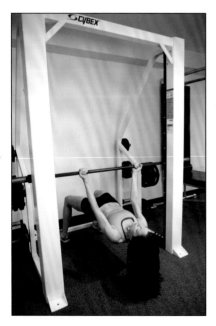

The Underhand Grip Bodyweight Row: Walk yourself under the bar and get into position. Pull up and arch your back. Try to touch the bar with your chest and then lower under control. 12 reps will do the trick and holding the top for 5 seconds each rep will increase the intensity in a big way!

2. Row Machine

This exercise is similar to what we just did, but we are going to opt for the neutral grip handles to be different from the last exercise. The neutral grip is where the palms of your hands face each other.

- Same deal here. Do your 12 rep max with 5 second holds at the top.

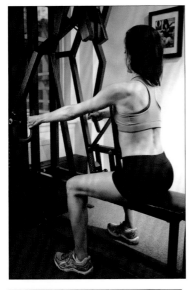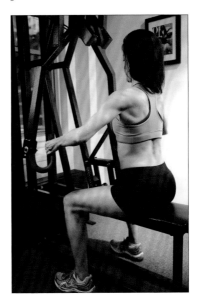

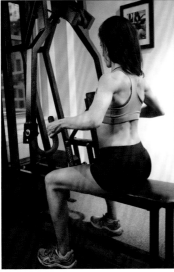

Make sure you hold the weight for 5 seconds in the contracted position. Well-defined back muscles are very sexy.

High Intensity Tip:
Remember not to swing or arch your back during the last few difficult reps. Poor form can result in injuries.

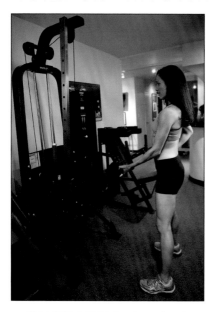 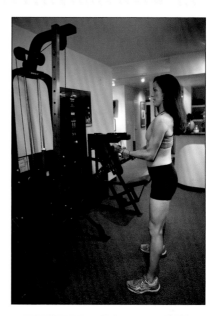

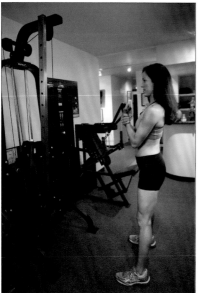 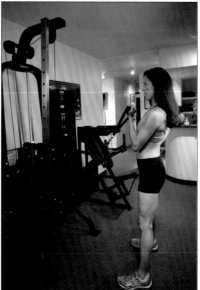

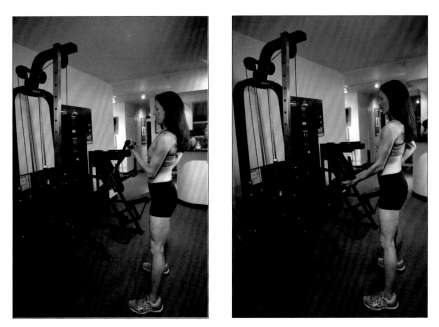

In this sequence you will lift with two hands and lower with one. Lower the weight in a slow and controlled fashion to get the most out of the exercise. One set for each arm is all that you'll need.

High Intensity Tip:

Add the High Intensity Cardio Kicker from Chapter Four to any of these workouts. By doing so, you'll still be finished and out the door in less than 30 minutes.

CHAPTER EIGHT:
HIGH INTENSITY REST

Let's face it, some of the greatest things that happen to me happen in my bed or on my couch: sleep and naps. You may be thinking, "but this is a workout book, why is he talking about sleep?" To get the best results from these workouts, you will need time to recover. The importance of a good, restful, and sound sleep in underrated. It is an equal part of a two part equation: the workout (or stimulation) and the recovery process. If either one of these components is not up to snuff, the whole program is not going to come close to giving you all that it can.

Here's the deal. Poor quality or lack of sleep has been linked to:

- Chronic Pain or Fibromyalgia
- Weight Gain
- Diabetes
- Heart Disease

It has also been recently linked to Alzheimer's disease. And this is just what we know about now. What other diseases do you think researchers will link poor sleep to? Don't take any chances; get a good night's sleep. If you have trouble sleeping, there are many options for you. Here are a few basic tips to try first.

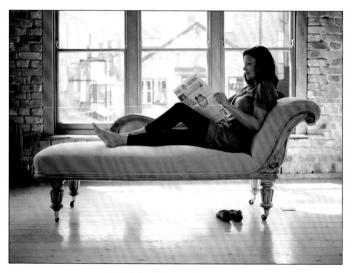

"Me" time is very important.

Reduce caffeine intake	You may want to start by cutting back from two cups a day to one, or possibly cutting out that afternoon cup. It could be the caffeine that you have in the afternoon or evening that is throwing you off. If that doesn't help, try switching to decaf for a while and see if that does the trick.
Don't eat chocolate at night	Dark chocolate is a healthy snack, but there is some caffeine in it, so it's best not to have any right before bed. Anytime one of my clients tells me they didn't sleep well the night before, I always ask if they ate chocolate before bed. Ninety percent of the time, the answer is "yes."
Avoid an "energy boost" after 8:00 p.m.	Sugar and sugary foods will give you an energy boost. That can be useful right before a workout, but not right before bed. If you were thinking about a big bowl of cereal before turning in for the night— FORGET IT! So what to do?

Eat foods high in magnesium	Ever get knocked out by an almond? Almonds are high in magnesium and may be just the thing to take the edge off and knock you out for the night. Since it's a much better snacking alternative than what you may have tried tonight, give it a shot. Other foods high in magnesium are legumes, pumpkin seeds, dark leafy green vegetables, and cashews.
Take a pill	Try something all natural, like L-Tryptophan or 5-HTP. These are basic, simple, and cost effective. So before you go buying some exotic concoction that doesn't even work as well, try these first.
Light reading	After you snack on some almonds and pop an L-Tryptophan capsule, how about a bedtime story to get you deep into an REM cycle? My favorite book about the benefits of sleep and the dangers of sleep deprivation is *Lights Out* by T.S. Wiley.

CHAPTER NINE:
HIGH INTENSITY NUTRITION

High Intensity Nutrition is just like these workouts: simple and right to the point. One of the reasons that people fail at dieting is that they don't know where to start. Even worse, they'll try an overly complicated one and get so overwhelmed that they quit before they begin. Remember, this book is for the person who is tight on time and high on stress. If you have all day to grow your own organic vegetables after gathering fresh eggs from your hens, I would imagine I don't need to offer any advice to you. The rest of us, however, need a simple, no-nonsense plan. If you have been following me on Twitter or Facebook, or read my book (*The 90-Second Fitness Solution*), you know that I'm a believer in eating "real" foods and always include whey protein in my diet.

The keys to a good nutrition program are simplicity and consistency. If you have no idea how many calories you are taking in or how much protein you're getting, how can you possibly know what changes you need to make? The first thing I do to get people on track is to get one meal at a time under control. These small changes will lead up to a big result and last much longer than going "all out" on a fad diet that will make you gain more weight than you lost after you bail on it.

Step One: Breakfast

While I'm sure you've heard it before, feeding your body properly first thing in the morning will set the tone (and your appetite) for the rest of the day. I have been promoting fresh vegetable juices with whey protein added or just a great tasting, high quality protein drink for many years. Make sure you focus on undenatured protein from New Zealand where grass-fed cows are being milked by season. To make this plan work, you will have to commit to having a protein drink for breakfast at least six out of seven days per week. Feel free to change flavors or spice up the shakes a little as long as you don't change the caloric intake very much. It will benefit you to know that you are getting the exact same amount of calories each morning and that it only took a few minutes to get the job done. You will have the choice of shaking these up with a shaker or making your shake in a blender so that you can throw in a banana or some frozen berries. Either way, get into the routine!

Not in the mood for a protein shake today? Try an egg white omelet loaded with veggies a few days per week. You can be creative with the veggie combinations that you use each time or stick with a recipe that you like and look forward to. Whatever you do, do not go for oatmeal or cereal for breakfast, as it will only add to your hips!

Step Two: Lunch

If you are like me, then you probably sit down to a relaxing three course meal for lunch at one of the finer restaurants in your area. Seriously, I'm moving like a freight train with no brakes all day. No time for a sit down. It's going to have to be quick and painless. I have two options for lunch that fit me best and will serve you as well, a monster salad or a second protein drink. Half of the week, I go across the street from work and get a chopped salad at the salad bar. You can't overdo fresh veggies so load up. Add a little protein like tuna, salmon, chicken, or egg whites and you have a complete meal. Where people go wrong is the dressing. Some of the dressing options have more calories than a steak dinner. Don't fall prey to this "big salad scam"—get sensible. Opt for a basic oil and vinegar (not too much) or my favorite—lemon juice. Again, the key is consistency, so try to stick with the same program more often than not.

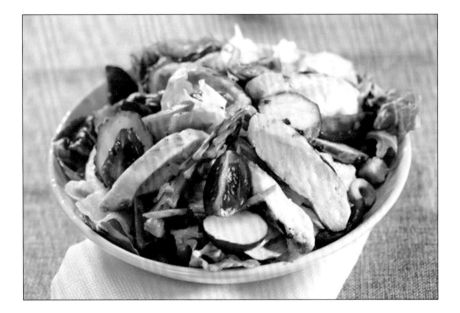

Option number two is a second protein drink. Whichever route you choose, stick with it for at least a month so you can see how the program is working before making adjustments. Another lunch option that I use each week is to have a Quinoa salad. Prepare the Quinoa over the weekend so you can simply scoop some into a bowl. Add chopped veggies along with some fresh parsley, cilantro, or basil. I usually add half of an avocado diced. Chopped walnuts or sunflower seeds optional. For a dressing:

2 Tbsp freshly squeezed lemon juice
2 Tbsp olive oil
1/4 tsp salt
Fresh ground pepper

The Grand Finale: Dinner

Last meal of the day can be disastrous if you aren't careful. Scenario one is where you starved yourself all day and the only thing you consumed was a sugary coffee-drink. This is bad. Your blood sugar levels are bouncing all around because you are living on high calorie caffeine with whipped cream all day, so the next meal you have will be converted to body fat since your body thinks it's starving. Scenario two is that 80 percent of your dinner consists of "the bread basket" and a nice chardonnay. I love the logic with scenario number two because people usually have dessert in this situation since they fell off their diet with the bread and wine. Keep it simple. Free range chicken or wild caught salmon with a vegetable and a salad is all you need. Remember that there are twenty-one meals in a week and you have to get twenty of them right to get rid of unwanted fat, so why not have a program laid out for you that lets you know exactly what to reach

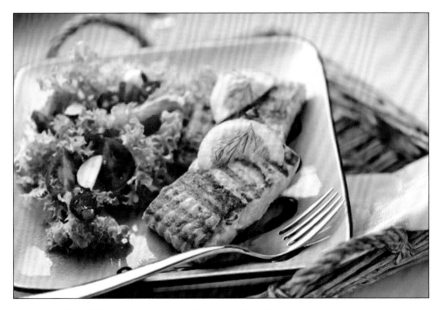

Grilled Salmon steak with fresh salad and balsamic vinegar sauce.

for when you are hungry? Well, I just did it for you. So try it, follow it, and embrace it! It will work, I promise.

The benefits of Grass Fed vs. Grain Fed:

Meat from grass-fed cattle is lower in artery-clogging saturated fat.

Grass-fed meat is higher in omega-3 fatty acids (Omega 3's are good for us and we want them).

Grass-fed meat is four times higher in vitamin E.

Last but not least, grass-fed meat is higher in conjugated linoleic acid (CLA), a nutrient associated with lower cancer risk and is also known to reduce bodyfat!

High Intensity Tip:
Whatever you choose for dinner whether it be chicken, fish, or beef make sure that the chicken and beef is grass fed and the fish is wild caught. This is very important to your health.

Snacks

Snacking in-between meals does not have to sabotage your diet. In fact, keeping your blood sugar levels balanced all day will help you stay on program. Some options would be a handful of nuts or a small piece of dark chocolate. Make sure that you eat something every three hours, whether it's a meal or a snack. I personally use one of many superfoods as my snacks. Superfoods are high nutrient foods that will satisfy your appetite while improving your health. Feel free to mix and match until you find the superfoods that will take the edge off. Remember portion control. Just because superfoods are a healthy snack, it doesn't mean you can eat as much as you want. A handful or a cup will do in most cases.

A short list of superfoods includes:

- Apples
- Avocado
- Blueberries
- Carrots
- Cherries
- Dark Chocolate
- Nuts (raw unsalted almonds and walnuts)
- Seeds (especially pumpkin and sunflower)
- Greek Yogurt

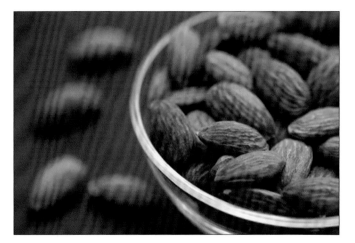

Raw almonds are a healthy snack that will keep you from reaching for the cookies.

Hydration

I know, I know, you think I'm going to tell you to drink some ridiculous amount of water each day. I'm not, so don't. When did we become this super hydrating, water consuming society? Drink and pee, drink and pee all day long. It's exhausting. If you're overheated and exercising too much, then I see the need for an increased amount of water. However, if you're following my program and getting your strength workouts in around 10 minutes, then you probably are not even sweating, so why would you need a gallon of water a day? I am 6'2" tall and weigh around 220 lbs. and I drink exactly one quart a day. No more, no less. If I feel dehydrated, I add a 16 ounce carton of coconut water to my schedule. Coconut water is high in potassium, which is very good for the body. It is necessary for the heart, kidneys, and other organs to work normally. We usually do not get adequate amounts of potassium in our diet, so getting it from coconut water is a great idea, as it will hydrate and give added potassium. I feel that there is the

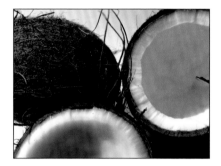

Coconut water is a great way to hydrate.

possibility of drinking too much water and that if you do, you will flush valuable nutrients out from your body. As you can see from my program and philosophy in general, I believe that "too much or too little" are no good. The goal is to get what you need. No more, no less.

CHAPTER TEN:
HIGH INTENSITY CLEANSING

I don't know about you, but in the past when I heard the word "cleansing," I cringed a bit. Why do I need to cleanse? I think I am "clean" enough: I eat pretty clean most of the time. Turns out I got it all wrong; let's see if you learn something new here as I did.

Generations ago, when our cows were still eating grass and hay, when our fruit and vegetables contained all the necessary nutrients, and our air and water did not include thousands of chemicals, impurities, poisons, and toxins, cleansing was not essential. Yet every ancient civilization has its ritual for cleansing, one which focuses on purification of mind and body. So why are we acting now that it is a new fad or an alien idea?

With increased amount of chemicals introduced into our life through water, air, soil, and food supply, our bodies get overwhelmed and our metabolism slows down. When this happens, reaching our health and weight loss goals is far from being a walk in the park. In fact, it's quite difficult to force the body to release a protective layer of fat when its own existence is being threatened by chemical substances. So which organs suffer the most and how do we prevent it from happening?

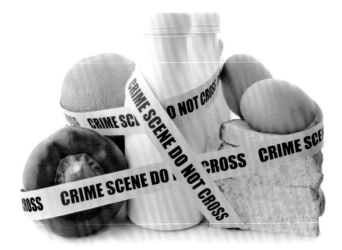

Just as your car has a filter and requires an oil change every 5,000 miles, just as your air conditioner has a filter and requires a replacement every a few months, so to your body has a filter, and it is called your liver. Keeping your filter (liver) clean and free of toxins is supposed to be happening naturally given the right conditions. What are the right conditions for liver cleansing? Ingesting and absorbing certain amino-acids, trace minerals, enzymes, and vitamins which unfortunately are not guaranteed nowadays due to the poor quality of food. As a result, our "self-cleaning" ability diminishes over the years, and our liver suffers from an overload. What happens then? Chemicals not captured by liver are being surrounded by a fat cell to protect the rest of the body from the possible damage. As we get exposed to more and more chemicals, our brain sends a signal to produce more and more fat cells as a survival mechanism. Please don't think that these chemicals wrapped up in fat can be dealt with by running a mile or doing burpees. It is not a logical solution and it doesn't work that way. People looking for better health and weight loss won't see the desired outcome until they do what? Until they CLEANSE and clean out that filter.

If done correctly, cleansing is a relatively simple procedure. It does not require hospitalization; it does not even require a day off work. If the proper tools are used, it's a process that will take no longer than 48 hours and will leave you feeling energized and feeling lighter. Oh, have I mentioned that it does not include frequent visits to the bathroom or uncomfortable cramps? Nope, not if you do it right, and let science and nature do its magic. The main purpose of the cleanse is to break down those fat cells, free up chemicals locked inside, and wash them out of the body. Is it simple? Yes. So let's not complicate things.

When I was first introduced to the idea of liver detoxification and deep nutritional cleanse, I really did not know what to expect. So just in case I prepared for the worst: I took a day off, locked myself in the room, and started feeling sorry for myself (just in case I felt bad). To my surprise, and almost disappointment, all I felt was bored and a little hungry; the rest was result of my imagination. After following a very simple protocol that focuses on flooding the body with nutrients and removing toxins from the liver, I released twelve pounds, and felt more energy than I had felt in years. I felt the difference, and I was hooked. I was now on a mission to share it with my family and friends, as I knew they all get exposed to the same elements, and in turn, they all could benefit from feeling more energy and numerous health benefits the body experiences when we "change the filter."

How would your life change if you could wake up before an alarm clock instead of hitting that snooze button five times? How would it even feel to have energy to play with kids after work instead of supporting that couch in the living room? What about self-image and self-esteem improvements when those last stubborn ten pounds are finally gone and you feel confident in that new swimming suit? All that and much more is possible, and in fact it is expected, as a "side effect" of a deep nutritional liver cleanse. Our bodies do work like well-oiled machines: lungs are helping us breathe without us thinking about it, the heart is pumping blood, and the temperature is being regulated within a tiny margin. Yet, sometimes it is our job to step in and support that vulnerable organism. Deep nutritional cleansing is one of those steps you can take to keep yourself healthy.

So is there a right and wrong way to do a liver cleanse? Oh yeah, there are plenty of opportunities for a major mess up, and here is what to watch out for:

- Make sure your body is ready for a cleanse, meaning that you have had proper nutrition and have an ample supply of amino-acids, enzymes, vitamins, and minerals required for a successful outcome

- Stay hydrated throughout the process. Remember, those toxins are being released from the liver and now need help to escape your body. Drinking plenty of water will ensure timely removal of the toxins.

- Do not cleanse for longer than 48 hours. Doing so can harm your body and be counterproductive. After 48 hours your body will switch into muscle-breaking-down mode instead of releasing fat and removing toxins.

- Doing a liver cleanse alone is no fun and will open you to making mistakes. Find a health-conscious friend who also cares about his or her quality of life, and do it together. Join a group that is doing an organized group cleanse or find a health professional to help with an initial health assessment to make sure your body is ready to cleanse

- Cleansing is not meant to treat any health conditions and should be used with caution. People who suffer from diabetes, take any medications or are recovering from surgery should check with their doctor or health practitioner first.

- And lastly, cleanse your liver every time you bring your car for an oil change or you bring your dog for teeth cleaning appointments. We do not stop living in a toxic world and being exposed to impurities so it makes sense to cleanse your liver periodically. "Lather, Rinse, Repeat." Well, you get the idea.

Conclusion

It is with great pleasure that I give to you *The High Intensity Fitness Revolution*. I hope the information provided will open your eyes to a new way of thinking about your health and fitness program.

Yours in Strength and Health,

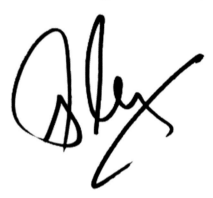

Pete Cerqua

SELECTED
BIBLIOGRAPHY

Adebamowo C.A., Cho E., Sampson L., Katan M.B., Spiegelman D., Willett W.C., Holmes M.D., "Dietary flavonols and flavonol-rich foods intake and the risk of breast cancer," International Journal of Cancer. 2005 Apr 20; 114(4):628-33.

Adebamowo C.A., Spiegelman D, Berkey C.S., Danby F.W., Rockett H.H., Colditz G.A., Willett W.C., Holmes M.D., "Milk consumption and acne in adolescent girls," Dermatology Online Journal. 2006 May 30; 12(4):1.

Adebamowo C.A., Spiegelman D., Danby F.W., Frazier A.L., Willett W.C., Holmes M.D., "High school dietary dairy intake and teenage acne," Journal of the American Academy of Dermatology. 2005 Feb; 52(2):207-14.

Anderson J.W., Hoie L.H., "Weight loss and lipid changes with low-energy diets: comparator study of milk-based versus soy-based liquid meal replacement interventions," Journal of the American College of Nutrition. 2005 Jun; 24(3):210-6.

Askling C., Karlsson J., Thorstensson A., "Hamstring injury occurrence in elite soccer players after preseason strength training with eccentric overload," Scandinavian Journal of Medicine Science and Sports. 2003 Aug; 13(4):244-50.

Audette J.F., Jin Y.S., Newcomer R., Stein L., Duncan G., Frontera W.R., "Tai Chi versus brisk walking in elderly women," Age Ageing. 2006 Jul; 35(4):388-93. Epub 2006 Apr 19.

Bandera E.V., Kushi L.H., Moore D.F., Gifkins D.M., McCullough M.L., "Consumption of animal foods and endometrial cancer risk: a systematic literature review and meta-analysis," Cancer Causes and Control 2007 Nov; 18(9):967-88. Epub 2007 Jul 19.

Barnett A., "Using recovery modalities between training sessions in elite athletes: does it help?" Sports Medicine. 2006; 36(9):781-96.

Bello N.T., Hajnal A., "Male rats show an indifference-avoidance response for increasing concentrations of the artificial sweetener sucralose," Nutrition Research 2005 Jul; 25(7):693-699.

Beneka A., Malliou P., Fatouros I., Jamurtas A., Gioftsidou A., Godolias G., Taxildaris K., "Resistance training effects on muscular strength of elderly are related to intensity and gender," Journal of Science Medicine in Sport. 2005 Sep; 8(3):274-83.

Bergstrom B.P., Cummings D.R., Skaggs T.A., "Aspartame decreases evoked extracellular dopamine levels in the rat brain: An in vivo voltammetry study," Neuropharmacology. 2007 Dec; 53(8):967-74. Epub 2007 Sep 29.

Berkey C.S., Rockett H.R., Willett W.C., Colditz G.A., "Milk, dairy fat, dietary calcium, and weight gain: a longitudinal study of adolescents," Archives of Pediatrics and Adolescent Medicine. 2005 Jun; 159(6):543-50.

Bigal M.E., Krymchantowski A.V., "Migraine triggered by sucralose--a case report," Headache. 2006 Mar; 46(3):515-7.

Bryner R.W., Ullrich I.H., Sauers J., Donley D., Hornsby G., Kolar M., Yeater R., "Effects of resistance vs. aerobic training combined with an 800 calorie liquid diet on lean body mass and resting metabolic rate," Journal of the American College Nutrition. 1999 Apr; 18(2):115-21.

Bulló M., Casas-Agustench P., Amigó-Correig P., Aranceta J., Salas-Salvadó J., "Inflammation, obesity and comorbidities: the role of diet," Public Health Nutrition. 2007 Oct; 10(10A):1164-72.

Carpinelli R.N., Otto R.M., "Strength training. Single versus multiple sets," Sports Medicine. 1998 Aug; 26(2):73-84.

Cauza E., Hanusch-Enserer U., Strasser B., Ludvik B., Metz-Schimmerl S., Pacini G., Wagner O., Georg P., Prager R., Kostner K., Dunky A., Haber P., "The relative benefits of endurance and strength training on the metabolic factors and muscle function of people with type 2 diabetes mellitus," Archives of Physical Medicine and Rehabilitation. 2005 Aug; 86(8):1527-33.

Chang J.C., Wu M.C., Liu I.M., Cheng J.T., "Increase of insulin sensitivity by stevioside in fructose-rich chow-fed rats," Hormone and Metabolic Research. 2005 Oct; 37(10):610-6.

Chan P., Tomlinson B., Chen Y.J., Liu J.C., Hsieh M.H., Cheng J.T., "A double-blind placebo-controlled study of the effectiveness and tolerability of oral stevioside in human hypertension," British Journal of Clinical Pharmacology. 2000 Sep; 50(3):215-20.

Chavarro J.E., Rich-Edwards J.W., Rosner B.A., Willett W.C., "A prospective study of dietary carbohydrate quantity and quality in relation to risk of ovulatory infertility," European Journal of Clinical Nutrition. 2007 Sep 19

Chavarro J.E., Rich-Edwards J.W., Rosner B.A., Willett W.C., "Dietary fatty acid intakes and the risk of ovulatory infertility," The American Journal of Clinical Nutrition. 2007 Jan; 85(1):231-7.

Chavarro J.E., Rich-Edwards J.W., Rosner B., Willett W.C., "A prospective study of dairy foods intake and anovulatory infertility," Human Reproduction (Oxford, England). 2007 May; 22(5):1340-7. Epub 2007 Feb 28.

Chiu H.F., Tsai S.S., Yang C.Y., "Nitrate in drinking water and risk of death from bladder cancer: an ecological case-control study in Taiwan," Journal of Toxicology and Environmental Health Part A. 2007 Jun; 70(12):1000-4.

Chiuve S.E, Giovannucci E.L., Hankinson S.E., Zeisel S.H., Dougherty L.W., Willett W.C., Rimm E.B., "The association between betaine and choline intakes and the plasma concentrations of homocysteine in women," The American Journal of Clinical Nutrition. 2007 Oct; 86(4):1073-1081.

Cho E., Chen W.Y., Hunter D.J., Stampfer M.J., Colditz G.A., Hankinson S.E., Willett W.C., "Red meat intake and risk of breast cancer among premenopausal women," Archives of Internal Medicine. 2006 Nov 13; 166 (20):2253-9.

Cho E., Seddon J.M., Rosner B., Willett W.C., Hankinson S.E., "Prospective study of intake of fruits, vegetables, vitamins, and carotenoids and risk of age-related maculopathy," Archives of Ophthalmology. 2004 Jun; 122 (6):883-92.

Christou M., Smilios I., Sotiropoulos K., Volaklis K., Pilianidis T., Tokmakidis S.P., "Effects of resistance training on the physical capacities of adolescent soccer players," Journal of Strength Conditioning Research 2006 Nov; 20(4):783-91

Davis J., Murphy M., Trinick T., Duly E., Nevill A., Davison G., "Acute effects of walking on inflammatory and cardiovascular risk in sedentary post-menopausal women," Journal of Sports Science. 2007 Oct 17; 1-7 [Epub ahead of print] .

Delagardelle C., Feiereisen P., Autier P., Shita R., Krecke R., Beissel J., "Strength/endurance training versus endurance training in congestive heart failure," Medicine and Science in Sports and Exercise. 2002 Dec; 34 (12):1868-72.

DiFrancisco-Donoghue J., Werner W., Douris .PC., "Comparison of once-weekly and twice-weekly strength training in older adults," British Journal of Sports Medicine. 2007 Jan; 41(1):19-22. Epub 2006 Oct 24.

Edworthy J., Waring H. "The effects of music tempo and loudness level on treadmill exercise," Ergonomics. 2006 Dec 15; 49(15):1597-610.

Fatouros I.G., Kambas A., Katrabasas I., Leontsini D., Chatzinikolaou A., Jamurtas A.Z., Douroudos I., Aggelousis N., Taxildaris K., "Resistance training and detraining effects on flexibility performance in the elderly are intensity-dependent," Journal of Strength Conditioning Research. 2006 Aug; 20(3):634-42.

Fatouros I.G., Taxildaris K., Tokmakidis S.P., Kalapotharakos V., Aggelousis N., Athanasopoulos S., Zeeris I., Katrabasas I., "The effects of strength training, cardiovascular training and their combination on flexibility of inactive older adults," International Journal of Sports Medicine. 2002 Feb; 23(2):112-9.

Fletcher I.M., Anness R., "The acute effects of combined static and dynamic stretch protocols on fifty-meter sprint performance in track-and-field athletes," Journal of Strength Conditioning Research. 2007 Aug; 21(3):784-7

Galvão D.A., Taaffe D.R., "Resistance exercise dosage in older adults: single- versus multiset effects on physical performance and body composition," Journal of the American Geriatric Society. 2005 Dec; 53(12):2090-7.

Herbert R.D., de Noronha M., "Stretching to prevent or reduce muscle soreness after exercise," Cochrane Database of Systematic Reviews (Online). 2007 Oct 17; (4):CD004577.

Herbert R.D., Gabriel M., "Effects of stretching before and after exercising on muscle soreness and risk of injury: systematic review," British Medical Journal. 2002 Aug 31; 325(7362):468.

Izquierdo M., Ibanez J, Gonzalez-Badillo J.J., Hakkinen K., Ratamess N.A., Kraemer W.J., French D.N., Eslava J., Altadill A, Asiain X., Gorostiaga E.M., "Differential effects of strength training leading to failure versus not to failure on hormonal responses, strength, and muscle power gains" Journal of Applied Physiology. 2006 May; 100(5):1647-56. Epub 2006 Jan 12.

Izquierdo M., Ibanez J., Hakkinen K., Kraemer W.J., Larrion J.L., Gorostiaga E.M., "Once weekly combined resistance and cardiovascular training in healthy older men," Medicine and Science in Sports and Exercise. 2004 Mar; 36(3):435-43.

Jones A.M., "Running economy is negatively related to sit-and-reach test performance in international-standard distance runners," International Journal of Sports Medicine. 2002 Jan; 23(1):40-3.

Kraemer W.J., Ratamess N.A., "Hormonal responses and adaptations to resistance exercise and training" Sports Medicine. 2005; 35(4):339-61.

Linnamo V., Pakarinen A., Komi P.V., Kraemer W.J., Hakkinen K., "Acute hormonal responses to submaximal and maximal heavy resistance and explosive exercises in men and women," Journal of Strength and Conditioning Research. 2005 Aug; 19(3):566-71.

Liu-Ambrose T., Khan K.M., Eng J.J., Janssen P.A., Lord S.R., McKay H.A., "Resistance and agility training reduce fall risk in women aged 75 to 85 with low bone mass: a 6-month randomized, controlled trial," Journal of the American Geriatric Society. 2004 May; 52(5):657-65.

Li Y., McClure P,W,, Pratt N., "The effect of hamstring muscle stretching on standing posture and on lumbar and hip motions during forward bending," Physical Therapy. 1996 Aug; 76(8):836-45; discussion 845-9.

Macone D., Baldari C., Zelli A., Guidetti L., "Music and physical activity in psychological well-being," Perceptual and Motor Skills. 2006 Aug; 103(1):285-95.

Mikesky A.E., Mazzuca S.A., Brandt K.D., Perkins S.M., Damush T., Lane K.A., "Effects of strength training on the incidence and progression of knee osteoarthritis," Arthritis and Rheumatism. 2006 Oct 15; 55(5):690-9.

Narloch J.A., Brandstater M.E., "Influence of breathing technique on arterial blood pressure during heavy weight lifting," Archives of Physical Medicine and Rehabilitation. 1995 May; 76(5):457-62.

Peate W.F., Bates G., Lunda K., Francis S., Bellamy K., "Core strength: a new model for injury prediction and prevention," Journal of Occupational Medicine and Toxicology. 2007 Apr 11; 2:3.

Pierson L.M., Herbert W.G., Norton H.J., Kiebzak G.M., Griffith P., Fedor J.M., Ramp W.K., Cook J.W., "Effects of combined aerobic and resistance training versus aerobic training alone in cardiac rehabilitation," Journal of Cardiopulmonary Rehabilitation. 2001 Mar-Apr; 21(2):101-10.

Rubin M.R,. Kraemer WJ, Maresh C.M., Volek J.S., Ratamess N.A., Vanheest J.L., Silvestre R., French D.N., Sharman M.J., Judelson D.A., Gomez A.L., Vescovi J.D., Hymer W.C., "High-affinity growth hormone binding protein and acute heavy resistance exercise," Medicine and Science in Sports and Exercise. 2005 Mar; 37(3):395-403.

Schmitz K.H., Ahmed R.L., Yee D., "Effects of a 9-month strength training intervention on insulin, insulin-like growth factor (IGF)-I, IGF-binding protein (IGFBP)-1, and IGFBP-3 in 30-50-year-old women," Cancer Epidemiology Biomarkers and Prevention. 2002 Dec; 11(12):1597-604.

Shrier I., "Does stretching improve performance? A systematic and critical review of the literature," Clinical Journal of Sports Medicine. 2004 Sep; 14(5):267-73.

Singh N.A., Clements K.M., Fiatarone M.A., "A randomized controlled trial of progressive resistance training in depressed elders," The Journals of Gerontology. Series A, Biological Sciences and Medical Sciences. 1997 Jan; 52(1):M27-35.

Smutok M.A., Reece C., Kokkinos P.F., Farmer C., Dawson .P, Shulman R., DeVane-Bell J., Patterson J., Charabogos C., Goldberg A.P., et al, "Aerobic versus strength training for risk factor intervention in middle-aged men at high risk for coronary heart disease," Metabolism: Clinical and Experimental. 1993 Feb; 42(2):177-84.

Stewart L.K., Flynn M.G., Campbell W.W., Craig B.A., Robinson J.P., Timmerman K.L., McFarlin B.K., Coen P.M., Talbert E., "The influence of exercise training on inflammatory cytokines and C-reactive protein," Medicine and Science in Sports and Exercise. 2007 Oct; 39(10):1714-9.

Stewart K.J., McFarland L.D., Weinhofer J.J., Cottrell E., Brown C.S., Shapiro E.P., "Safety and efficacy of weight training soon after acute myocardial infarction," Journal of Cardiopulmonary Rehabilitation. 1998 Jan-Feb; 18(1):37-44.

Szabo A,, Small A., Leigh M., "The effects of slow- and fast-rhythm classical music on progressive cycling to voluntary physical exhaustion," Journal of Sports Medicine and Physical Fitness. 1999 Sep; 39(3):220-5.

Westcott W.L., La Rosa Loud R,, Cleggett E,, Glover S,, "Effects of Regular and Slow Speed Training on Muscle Strength," Journal of Sports Medicine and Physical Fitness. 2001 Jun; 41(2):154-8.

Westcott W.L., La Rosa Loud R., Glover S., "Strength Training Frequency," unpublished study available at http://www.ssymca.org/quincy/westcott/research_studies.html.

Yamashita S., Iwai K., Akimoto T, Sugawara J., Kono I., "Effects of music during exercise on RPE, heart rate and the autonomic nervous system," The Journal of Sports Medicine and Physical Fitness. 2006 Sep; 46(3):425-30.

ACKNOWLEDGMENTS

This book would not be possible if it were not for the love, support, and friendship of some very special people in my life:

Pete Cerqua

Marylou Cerqua and Pete Cerqua, Sr.
A.k.a. Mom and Dad. Thank you for laying the groundwork and foundation of morals and principles that helped me build a business and raise a son. I love you both very much.

Gregg Stebben
Thank you for your friendship. You are the person that got the ball rolling on this book and opened doors for me. Whether you are on the east coast or west coast, it's nice to know you are close by.

Tony Lyons
I am honored to be a Skyhorse author. Thank you for the opportunity to be a part of the fastest growing independent publishing house in America and welcoming me to the Skyhorse family.

Jason Katzman
Thank you for your guidance and wisdom, without which this book would not be possible.

Cora Poage
Take a High Intensity workout and add beauty and grace. That's what you bring to the table. Thank you for making the exercises look good. But most importantly, your open mind to a different health and fitness approach.

Dara Jewett (photographs)

Thank you for taking my vision and making it visible for all to see. Your flexibility, professionalism, and artistic design are unmatched. darajewett.com

The Gym Source

Friends for over twenty years! Thanks to Rich Miller and Nigel Anderson for letting us shoot at your NYC flagship location. When I met you both in 1988, you had a desk for each of you, a small showroom, and one location. Twenty-four years and thirty locations later, you are the gold standard for home and gym exercise equipment. I am proud to know you both.

90-Second Fitness Trainers

I am very fortunate to be working with close friends on a daily basis: Corrie Blissit, Mike Pinto, Nedezda Karlina, Nick Westmeyer, Annette Nack. All masters at their craft and great sounding boards. Thank you.

Victoria Toujilina

Thank you for being a part of this project and a part of my life. Your attention to detail combined with a love for the subject takes this work to the next level. Remember when we talked about writing a book together? We just did. Here's to many more books.

Our Tribe

When reading the different interpretations that define the word tribe, I can't help but think this word best describes our extended family. Surrounding ourselves with "like-minded" people while distancing us from the negative energy commonly found on a daily basis is what makes our tribe the fun, motivated and life loving group that we are. As we continue to move forward together, please remember the immortal words of David

Bowie—"Let's Dance." Paula Penna, Frank and Tish Jurgens, Bob and Denise Scully, Cindy Clark, Heather Sica-Leonard, Maggie Carchrie and Thomas Leigh, Nancy Leduc, Kim and Mike Johnson, Vicky and George Honour, Lora Congelosi, Rachel Penna-Scheer, Chandler Fann, Cindy Koltz, Jennifer Mikol, Gregory Cohen, Wendy Coleman, Cynthia Zingler, Boo Fuqua, Nicole Hudson, Kay Bollmus, and Jennifer Ward.

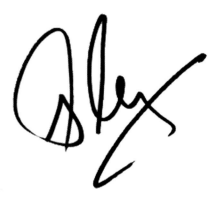

Victoria Toujilina

Pete Cerqua

It is such an honor to be a part of this project with you. I used to hate weight lifting and high intensity until you came along. You showed me how to get stronger and healthier in less time than it takes to make a bed. I loved working on this book together, and I look forward to more opportunities to collaborate.

Ilya Minarov

It is not often we see young people being so focused and determined to make the most out of this life. I feel so privileged to call you my son, to watch you grow and become such an intelligent and independent young man. Thank you for always believing in me and inspiring me to believe in myself. And Ilya? We don't get lost, we always know where we are and where we are going.